# The Neuropsychology of written Language Disorders:

## diagnosis and intervention

Steven G. Feifer, Ed.S., NCSP     Philip A. De Fina, Ph.D., ABPdN

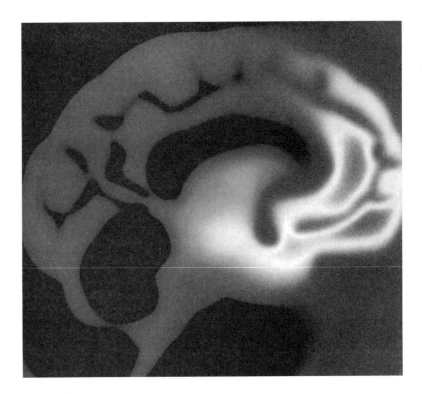

contributing authors

Mary Joann Lang, Ph.D., ABPN

Frances McCreary Holland, Ph.D

Cheryl H. Coughlin, OTR/L

Foreword by Cecil R. Reynolds, Ph.D., ABPN, ABPP

The Neuropsychology of Written Language Disorders: Diagnosis and Intervention Workbook by Steven G. Feifer and Philip A. De Fina; foreword by Cecil R. Reynolds.

Published by School Neuropsych Press, LLC
PO Box 413
Middletown, MD 21769
Snpress@frederickmd.com

Cover designed by Susan Hough of Octavo Designs in Frederick, Maryland.
All illustrations courtesy of Mark Burrier of Octavo Designs in Frederick, Maryland.

ISBN# 0-9703337-1-4

Printed in the United States of America

# ACKNOWLEDGMENTS

Any scholarly endeavor attempting to explain and rationalize the human brain requires the prudent work ethic and collective talents of numerous brains. A special thanks to Dr. Amy Gabel of the Psychological Corporation, as well as Dr. Scott Bishop of Riverside Publishing, for their sound advice and thoughtful commentary on tests and measurement issues. A very special thanks to Susan Hough and Mark Burrier from Octavo Designs for their creative minds and kindred spirit in seeing this project through to fruition. Much appreciation to Joseph E. Gorga for his continued support and words of encouragement during trying times, as well as a heartfelt thanks to Jennifer Kerr of Lord Sterling Schools, for providing much needed administrative assistance. In addition, the secretarial support of Irene M. Seitz was most appreciated. A very special thank you to our friend and colleague Robert Jacobs, for being the glue which held this project together. As always, we tip our hats to the brilliant minds of the many researchers, scholars, philosophers, and neuroscientists who continue to shape and influence our conceptualization of learning and behavior in children through their dedicated pursuit to fully comprehend life's greatest mystery; namely, the human brain.

Lastly, a special thank you to the teachers and administration at Dr. Charles R. Drew Elementary School in Montgomery County, Maryland including Eileen Evans, principal and Jennifer Huff, special education coordinator. Much appreciation to the following teachers for providing writing samples from their students for this book: Melissa Fean (1st), Susan Little (2nd), Wanda O'Neale (3rd), Linda Dunnigan (4th), Amy Holland (5th) and Kim Leichtling (5th/GT).

## DEDICATION

*"To Darci, whose love I cherish and whose devotion I envy."* - SGF

*"To my parents, Joe and Camille, for their never ending support and encouragement in all of my professional endeavors. Their love and wisdom has guided me throughout my life."* - PAD

| Steven G. Feifer, Ed.S., NCSP    Philip A. De Fina, Ph.D., ABPdN

# table of contents

## FOREWARD

Writing is an often overlooked area in many aspects of neuropsychology but also in school psychology. Writing is a particular form of expressive language that requires the coordination of multiple jointly working brain structures for successful completion. It is thus clearly a neuropsychological function and one that falls in the expressive domain. While motor functions and accompanying disturbances of fine motor control as well as difficulties with visual motor integration can create great difficulties in some aspects of written expression, these are not true disorders of written language and so must be distinguished as various forms of dyspraxia. Feifer and De Fina in this concise treatise have provided a succinct treatment of the neuropsychological foundations and development of written language from both the viewpoint of normal developmental phenomena as well as issues surrounding what can go wrong. They distinguish various forms of written language problems and trace their functional neuroanatomic roots for us. In a succinct manner, they have provided the experienced clinician with a ready reference to the neuropsychology of written language that accents the practical needs of the clinician.

The work is particularly strong in providing remedial strategies that are steeped in an experiential basis for the learner. Indeed, this is quite appropriate as written language is an involved task that requires experience and action as opposed to passive remedial approaches associated with common instructional practices. Motivation is addressed (as it should be) as motivational constraints are one of the major barriers to overcoming deficiencies in written language. Thus, in a clear and concise manner, Feifer and De Fina have provided the knowledgeable clinician with a ready reference manual that will assist in differential diagnosis of written language disorders along with motor disturbances and guidelines with practical examples for the provision of remedial services. Such a succinct treatment is needed in the field and will be useful to those who work with such children. The clinician who is new to written language disorders will need to acquire more extensive background and training to achieve the full benefit of Feifer and De Fina's insights and instruction but should come back to this work as they approach journeyman status.

Those who are unacquainted with neuropsychological approaches to written language disorders will find the work helpful as well since clearly brain function is involved at every level of written language. Neuropsychological models have much to offer not only in understanding the basis for a child's specific disturbance in written language but also in the development of remedial approaches that match the component of deficiency seen in the child's efforts. This is in fact one of the great strengths of neuropsychological approaches and one that Feifer and De Fina obviously appreciate. Though some may disagree with their treatment of intelligence testing and current diagnostic standards, this work should be a welcome addition to the libraries of school psychologists and other diagnosticians who encounter children and adolescents who fall at any point on the continuum of written language disorders.

Cecil R. Reynolds, PhD, ABPN, ABPP
Bastrop, TX
February, 2002

# overview of written Language

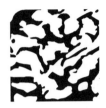

## Chapter 1

"An author hates to write, but loves having written."
— oscar madison

Trepidation, fear, anxiety, angst. Perhaps no other school endeavor entails more apprehensive feelings and emotions than a timed independent written language activity. By most standards, the quintessential feature of successful learning revolves around the proficiency and competency of a student's reading and written language skills. Students are expected to write in a variety of styles, employing *narrative, informative*, or *persuasive* skills while simultaneously demonstrating their linguistic prowess through their mastery of spelling, syntax, grammar, capitalization, punctuation and organization of ideas. In essence, the ability to echo thought in a cohesive manner through symbolic representation has been an academic focus and barometer for educational success since the dawning of formalized instruction. Written language is tantamount to a communal memory system that taps the wisdom, insights, and knowledge of previous generations. As Sagan (1980) noted:

> *"Writing is perhaps the greatest of human inventions, binding together people, citizens of distant epochs, who never knew each other. Books break the shackles of time, and inspire us to make our own contributions to the collective knowledge of the human species," (Cosmos, p. 232)*

The recent evolution of written language in human beings manifested itself nearly five thousand years ago in Western Asia as **Cuneiform Writing**, antedating the use of alphabets by some three thousand years. This type of writing utilized wedge-shaped strokes, inscribed primarily in clay or stone, that were used primarily as a means for transcribing economic trades and transactions. The scribe would start at the top left edge of the tablet, work downward to the bottom edge, then return to the top of the next column in a row-like fashion similar to a modern newspaper. Our current alphabet system, a derivative of the Roman alphabet, originated thousands of years ago in Greece, though lowercase letters were not used until after the 8th century. Prior to the invention of movable type in 1450, there were perhaps tens of thousands of books in Europe, all of which were handwritten. Fifty years later, there were more than ten million books available. Today, the great libraries of the world contain trillions of bits of information in words, so that if one book were read per week, approximately one tenth of one percent would be read in a lifetime. Notwithstanding, the number of new books grows exponentially each year.

For decades, written language has been given increased emphasis among contemporary educators, although some may argue that writing deficiencies are not awarded the legitimacy of reading or math disabilities (Sandler, et. al., 1992). For instance, most remedial and tutorial educational programs in elementary schools consist of reading-based interventions such as Title 1, Reading Recovery, Targeted Reading Intervention, and Alphabetic Phonics instruction, which all emphasize reading as opposed to written language skills. Our current political agenda has decreed that schools should strive for all students to be reading on grade level by the fourth grade, though little mention has been made of written language prowess. Within the world of math and science, there has always been much competition with the foreign elite to determine bragging rights for the technological sophistication of a given culture. Nevertheless, with the advent of word processing, spell-checks, grammar-checks, and even hand-held Franklin desktop spellers, technology has de-emphasized the need for exacting paper and pencil composition. Letter writing has become a lost art, replaced by e-mail correspondence, while accurate spelling has been trivialized by the power of a microchip. In fact, most standardized tests of written language skills are often insensitive to the subtle nuances of grammar, fluency, and syntax, instead over-relying on spelling aptitude, handwriting clarity, and punctuation skills. Additionally, a recent survey of fine-motor activity requirements in elementary schools in Massachusetts showed that 30% to 60% of classroom time on written language was devoted primarily to handwriting skills, leaving limited portions of the day for actual linguistic instruction to commence (Deuel, 1995). Since writing is the last language skill to develop ontogenetically, after comprehension, speech, and reading (Sandler, et. al, 1992), most written language disabilities are likely to persist into secondary school as well. Therefore, a great paradox exists between the amount of time, emphasis, and instructional breadth involved in teaching the taxonomy of written expression at earlier ages versus the increased written demands confronting students at the secondary level. Consequently, most remedial assistance in written language takes place within a special education setting where specific Individualized Instructional Plans are crafted to meet the needs of a child. As depicted in Table 1-1, various aspects of the written language process need to be introduced as early as preschool, with each subsequent developmental stage requiring additional elaboration and synthesis of both motor and linguistic capabilities.

By the time children have reached 1st grade, they should have developed a relative mastery of articulatory, syntactic, semantic, and pragmatic features of spoken language (Bailet, 2001). What awaits is a linguistic marathon of sorts, chalked with abstractions and syllogisms, and tempered with devilishly cunning linguistic twists and turns. In essence, a second order symbol-system must now be mastered. One that associates the sequences of the 26 letter formations with some 80,000 meaningful words in the English language, which can be arranged to form an infinite array of conceptual thoughts and knowledge bases emanating from the human mind. The ultimate quest in this communicative adventure is to learn to write, so that writing can become a means for learning. In other words, students ultimately need to use written language as a method of reasoning, problem solving, and persuasion. At its highest level, written language truly is an art, a majestic symphony of words that paint a portrait of our souls, capable of capturing the human spirit with prosaic elegance unparalleled by no other species.

The human brain has built-in mechanisms to ensure that neurolinguistic skills are preserved at all cost. The plasticity associated with the brain in light of injury reflects the notion that there are inherent back-up systems in place if the cortical language centers become compromised. Since written expression is the last linguistic skill to develop in children, the effect of early brain lesions may not be reflected in discrete language disturbances until much later in childhood, when more higher-level linguistic skills emerge. In essence, children actually grow into their deficit patterns a by-product of faulty neurodevelopment, whether by disease or trauma.

## TABLE 1-1

| Developmental stages of writing | |
|---|---|
| stage | characteristics |
| 1. **Imitation** (preschool to first grade) | • Attempts to mimic true writing<br>• Awareness of spatial arrangement of letter groups (words)} and of lines<br>• Acquisition of letter and number formations<br>• Beginning appreciation of spelling accuracy and use of invented spellings |
| 2. **Graphic Presentation** (first & second grades) | • Finger play songs, drawing, painting form boards to develop fine-motor dexterity<br>• Preoccupation with visual appearances<br>• Discovery of conventions of capitalization, punctuation, and sentence structure<br>• Increasingly precise and distal fine-motor regulation<br>• Rapid increase in spelling ability<br>• Use of unsophisticated language |
| 3. **Syntactic Incorporation** (late second to fourth grade) | • Awareness of writing as a synthetic process<br>• Integration of conventions (punctuation, capitalization) with language (morphology, syntax, narrative organization)<br>• Written language less sophisticated than speech<br>• Little emphasis on well-planned writing<br>• Awareness of spatial formats (paragraphs, letters)<br>• Start of cursive writing |
| 4. **Automatization** (fourth to seventh grade) | • Writing with less expenditure of conscious effort<br>• Growing capacity to write and think<br>• Increased note-taking skills<br>• Proofing, editing, and rewriting text<br>• Ability to produce larger volumes of writing<br>• Written language approximates speech |

Steven G. Feifer, Ed.S., NCSP   Philip A. De Fina, Ph.D., ABPdN

| stage | characteristics |
|---|---|
|  | • Greater stress on planning and draft writing<br>• Early development of report and expository writing and research skills |
| 5. **Elaboration**<br>(seventh to ninth grade) | • Writing used to establish and express a viewpoint<br>• Written language exceeds complexity of everyday speech<br>• Problem solving and idea development occur through writing<br>• Summarization through writing becomes a common task<br>• Organization and use of information from multiple sources<br>• Extensive use of transitions and cohesive ties (words such as finally, for example, therefore, or but) |
| 6. **Abstractions and Personalizations**<br>(ninth grade and beyond) | • Development of individual writing styles<br>• Use of different writing styles and formats appropriate to subject matter and purpose (lab reports, research papers, expository essays, poetry)<br>• Greater variation of language use<br>• Sophistication of vocabulary and use of figurative language, irony, symbolism<br>• Writing as a medium for experimentation<br>• Writing as a method of reasoning, problem solving, and persuasion |

\* Adapted from Levine, M.D., & Reed, M., (1999). *Developmental Variation and Learning Disorders*. Massachusetts: Educators Publishing Service, Inc. (p.349).

Unfortunately, there is little evidence to suggest that written language proficiency among students is increasing, while there is mounting evidence that special education interventions for written language disabilities have minimal impact on disabled students. In fact, this is especially true when diagnosis and intervention are delayed. The National Center for Educational Statistics (1999) long term writing assessment report focused on changes and/or trends in writing mechanics and fluency that have occurred between

1984 and 1996. An analysis of writing mechanics sampled 500 essays from Grades 4, 8, and 11 and measured attributes such as sentence length and average number of sentences per passage. In addition, each passage was evaluated using a six-point holistic scoring system on fluency attributes such as spelling and grammar, elaboration of ideas, and organization and clarity. A synopsis of Table 1-2 is as follows:

- On average in 1996 papers, two overall measures usually associated with improvement in writing skills (average number of full words per paper and average number of sentences per paper) increased when compared to performance in 1984. Increases were at grades 8 and 11 only.

- Average number of words per sentence showed no change between 1984 and 1996.

- Even though 8th and 11th graders' papers were longer in 1996, their error rates (average number of all errors per 100 words) did not change from 1984 to 1996.

While the results of this national longitudinal study show minimal, if any, measurable increase in written language skills over the past decade, there has been little supporting evidence of the efficacy of special education in remediating written language disorders in children. The most widely accepted paradigm for diagnosing reading and written language disabilities in children relies heavily on discrepancies between a student's cognitive ability and current levels of academic achievement. Hence, the average age at which a child is classified as being learning disabled is 9 years old, or 3rd grade, since this is when discrepancies become most prevalent (Shaywitz, 1998). The controversial presumption that psychological tests can cleanly and indisputably measure just intelligence, while other tests can cleanly and indisputably measure a specific academic endeavor, remains problematic. Consequently, there are numerous pitfalls inherent within this psychometrically unsound criterion for the identification of learning disabilities in children.

Steven G. Feifer, Ed.S., NCSP    Philip A. De Fina, Ph.D., ABPdN

## TABLE I — 2

### NAEP Trends in writing

overall characteristics of papers: 1984 and 1996

THE NATION'S REPORT CARD
## NAEP

| Mechanics Measure | Grade | Year | Overall Average | Holistic Scores 1,2,3 Lower half of scale | 4,5,6 Upper half of scale |
|---|---|---|---|---|---|
| Average number of full words per paper | 4 | 1996 | 35.4 | 28.4 | 53.9 |
| | | 1984 | 33.8 | 27.9 | 47.7 |
| | 8 | 1996 | 79.4* | 59.2* | 104.2* |
| | | 1984 | 67.5 | 51.1 | 89.5 |
| | 11 | 1996 | 104.4* | 68.6 | 124.4 |
| | | 1984 | 93.3 | 62.0 | 115.0 |
| Average number of sentences per paper | 4 | 1996 | 2.6 | 2.1 | 3.9 |
| | | 1984 | 2.6 | 2.2 | 3.6 |
| | 8 | 1996 | 5.2* | 3.8 | 6.8* |
| | | 1984 | 4.4 | 3.4 | 5.8 |
| | 11 | 1996 | 6.5* | 4.1 | 7.8* |
| | | 1984 | 5.6 | 3.7 | 6.9 |
| Average number of words per sentence | 4 | 1996 | 16.1 | 16.1* | 16.0 |
| | | 1984 | 15.1 | 14.3 | 16.8 |
| | 8 | 1996 | 17.7 | 18.3 | 16.9 |
| | | 1984 | 17.3 | 17.5 | 17.0 |
| | 11 | 1996 | 18.2 | 18.8 | 17.7 |
| | | 1984 | 18.2 | 18.8 | 17.7 |
| Average number of all errors per 100 words | 4 | 1996 | 17.2 | 19.2 | 11.8 |
| | | 1984 | 15.5 | 17.1 | 11.6 |
| | 8 | 1996 | 10.2 | 12.1 | 7.9 |
| | | 1984 | 9.2 | 10.3 | 7.7 |
| | 11 | 1996 | 7.4 | 9.2 | 6.3 |
| | | 1984 | 7.0 | 8.4 | 6.0 |

*Statistically significant difference from 1984, at the 95-percent certainty level.

Notwithstanding, given the over-reliance on the aptitude/achievement paradigm, most children are identified as needing assistance far too late in their academic careers, thereby squandering critical learning windows of opportunity in which foundation skills can be mastered (Feifer & De Fina, 2000). Perhaps this is why 74 percent of children identified as being learning disabled by 3rd grade remain in special education through 9th grade (Lyon, 1996). In summary, it would appear that both regular education students and special education students need assistance in the foundation, development, and implementation of an extremely elusive craft - namely, written expressive skills.

# shortcomings of intelligence Tests

# Chapter 2

*"we shouldn't ask how smart are you? But rather how are you smart?"*
*— Howard Gardner*

The evolution of intelligence test measurement has not necessarily followed the basic Darwinian principles and tenets of selective behavioral adaptation over time, as has the evolution of intelligence itself. For instance, human beings themselves have evolved from fear-ridden cave dwellers to mammals capable of domesticating fires, inventing tools, developing a symbolic communication system, and grasping the physical laws of the universe. In other words, the evolution of intelligence can be observed not just in the exponential growth of our technologically oriented culture, but also in the manner in which human beings respond intuitively with reason and insight. At the turn of the twentieth century, intelligent Americans were choosing a wide variety of careers, not necessarily limited to traditional 'white-collar' occupations. In fact, in 1900 more than two-thirds of the presidents and chairmen of America's largest corporations did not have a college degree (Herrnstein & Murray, 1994). When colleges opened their doors to educate more students throughout the twentieth century, America began to evolve from an industrial-based society toward a more technologically based culture. Today, we find ourselves at the forefront of an increasingly sprawling communications-based society fueled and ignited by computer technology.

Throughout this mercurial era, psychologist James Flynn noted that intelligence test scores were on the rise, by as much as one quarter point per year (Herrnstein & Murray, 1994). Certainly, plausible factors for the upward mobility of intelligence test scores include improvements in public education, health care, and nutrition, though the rigors and demands of a culture valuing intellectual thought over physical brawn have also helped to fuel this cognitive uprise of some 7-10 points per generation. Therefore, the evolutionary pattern of intelligence suggests that over time an evolving set of intellectual clusters, knowledge, skills, and abilities considered valuable by society have been reinforced, while groups of intellectual traits that carry little adaptive value have been discarded.

Nevertheless, the science of measuring human cognitive functioning has not necessarily followed this natural selection process. In other words, the measurement of intelligence has stalled somewhat in its evolution, falling prey to the popular assumption that the dynamic property of the human brain - and its capacity to arrange some 100 billion neurons interfacing with some 30 trillion synapses - can be quantified by a single numeric score. The daunting task of measuring higher cortical functioning and abstract reasoning skills has been at the forefront of cognitive psychology since the end of the nineteenth century. Initially, Alfred Binet and Theodore Simon worked to develop specific methods in France to unlock the mystery behind various mental functions. Their research focused on higher mental processes instead of simple sensory functions as postulated by some of their predecessors (Sattler, 1988). With the introduction of the Binet-Simon Scales, the testing movement began to flourish in the United States. Perhaps of greater significance was Lewis Terman's revision of the initial Binet-Simon Scale, and the adoption of the term *Intelligence Quotient (IQ)*, by dividing mental age scores by chronological age.

However, it was David Wechsler, whose search for a global nature of intelligence during World War I, lead to the systemic selection of 11 subtests which have come to dominate the field. Although its theoretical construct was crafted seventy-five years ago, the Wechsler Intelligence Scale for Children, now in its third edition, still remains the single most popular measure among psychologists in the assessment of children. The Wechsler concept of intelligence, with its simplistic dichotomy depicting verbal versus nonverbal problem skills, has become entrenched and optimized in the pop-psychology market, particularly with respect to psychoeducational testing in the school system. In fact, the notion of a verbal intelligence quotient versus a nonverbal intelligence quotient continues to have mass popular appeal among educators, even in the absence of any empirically based support from factor analytical models (McGrew, 1994). Indeed,

Wechsler originally intended simply to organize a test for both English and non-English speaking soldiers to allow for the expression of intelligence. Consequently, a set of nonverbal problem solving tasks were created to evaluate the cognitive skills of soldiers not well versed in the English language.

During the second half of the 20th century, computer oriented technology spawned the advent of factor analytical constructs to measure various strands of cognition. Furthermore, the use of neuroimaging devices to detect brain functioning has exploded, and the notion of multiple intelligences coupled with the artificial intelligence mediums has evoked more sophisticated and insightful methods of quantifying intellectual prowess. However, the evolution of intelligence test measurement has not necessarily coincided with these new theoretical models of cognition, due in part to the intuitive appeal of representing higher cortical functioning with a single numeric score.

The mass reluctance of practicing psychologists to loosen their hold on the outdated Wechsler paradigm has drawn siege and discontent from many in the field. Howard Gardner has been especially critical (1999), claiming that the parochialism of the Western view of intelligence has ignored traits highly valued in other cultures such as obedience, moral fiber, and good listening skills. Hence, Gardner has argued for a *multiple intelligences* model focusing on traits and abilities including logical-mathematical intelligence, linguistic intelligence, spatial intelligence, musical intelligence, bodily-kinesthetic intelligence, interpersonal intelligence, and intrapersonal intelligence. As Gardner (1985) noted:

> *"Much of the information probed for in intelligence tests reflects knowledge gained from living in a specific social and educational milieu. For instance, the ability to define "tort" or to identify the author of the "Iliad" is highly reflective of the kind of school one attends or the taste's of one's family. In contrast, intelligence tests rarely assess skills in assimilating new information or in solving new problems. This bias towards crystallized intelligence rather than fluid knowledge can have astounding consequences. An individual can lose his entire frontal lobes, in the process of becoming a radically different person, unable to display any initiative or to solve new problems, yet may continue to exhibit an IQ close to genius level. Moreover, the intelligence test reveals little about a an individual's potential for future growth or how the mind works." (Frames of Mind, p.18)*

Factor analytic models of intelligence, which use a set of statistical procedures to analyze the intercorrelations or covariances among a set of variables, have also argued against a single, unitary intelligence model of human cognitive abilities (McGrew, 1994).

Using an impressive set of statistical evidence and meta-cognitive analysis covering 50 years worth of cognitive data, Carroll (1993) deduced 69 narrow band cognitive abilities, best conceptualized by eight cognitive factors: Fluid Intelligence, Crystallized Intelligence, General Memory and Learning, Visual Perception, Auditory Perception, Retrieval Ability, Cognitive Speed, and Processing Speed. These independent knowledge sources were thought to account for the range of attributes that comprise human cognitive functioning. At the apex of this hierarchical model lies a general intelligence factor or (g), which represents an underlying general intellectual ability that presumably is the basis for most intellectual behavior (McGrew, 1994). Unlike Gardner's theory of multiple intelligences, these cognitive constructs have been operationalized into a single cognitive battery; namely the **Woodcock-Johnson III**. The test was revised in the fall of 2000, and whether its sophisticated constructs supported by empirical data will supplant the simplistic dichotomy of the Wechsler series measures remains to be seen. Nevertheless, the *Woodcock-Johnson III* makes a concerted effort to examine the various domains of cognition in a comprehensive manner by taking a multiple factor view of human intelligence, not necessarily relying on a single unitary score.

While statisticians may ponder over the significance of factor loadings with respect to human intellectual functioning, and sociologists may squabble over the relative definitions of *intelligence* as dictated by the demands of a given culture, the field of neuropsychology has directed its acumen toward the organ accountable for all human endeavors: the brain. The discipline of neuropsychology has gained massive appeal by recapturing the science side of psychology, directing its study of cognition towards brain-behavioral relations. Of particular interest for most educators is the integration of school-based learning with specific neural constructs that lay the foundation for the acquisition of reading, math, and written language skills. According to A.R. Luria, considered by most to be the founder of modern-day neuropsychology, the brain consists of three processing blocks that channel information. Stated simply, there lies

1) an arousal-activation stage consisting of brain structures in the reticular activation regions or brain stem,

2) a perceptual integration stage housed in the anterior cortical regions of the brain,

3) and an executive functioning stage located in the frontal lobes (Goldberg, 1990).

In Luria's terms, a behavior or trait is the product or interaction of many cognitive elements, each mediated by a different brain structure. Thus, a neuropsychological model of cognition based upon functional units was created to evaluate cognitive, linguistic, and sensorimotor functions (Lezak, 1995). This notion of functional units or systems, with different cerebral representations, contrasts harshly with the simplistic notion of one-on-one brain mapping that had come to dominate the field. However, Luria's theories are somewhat incomplete, as he focused most of his efforts on the explorations of left hemispheric functioning only. According to Goldberg (1990), Luria's main interests were in language and the interface between culture and cognition. Consequently, his scholarly work on the contributions of the right hemisphere with respect to higher cortical functions was somewhat limited. Still, the work of Luria has been at the forefront of most information processing theories of intelligence.

Many noteworthy efforts have been made toward operationalizing Luria's basic tenets into user-friendly assessment instruments, including Charlie Golden's Luria-Nebraska battery, as well as Alan Kaufman's Kaufman Assessment Battery for Children (K-ABC), published in 1983. Though an ardent supporter of the Wechsler Intelligence Scales, Kaufman (1994) acknowledged that psychologists tend to over-rely on full scale scores, displaying an inherent bias in their belief that human cognitive functioning can be represented in a single numeric score, and fail to account for the test's limitations as indicated in Table 2-1. In fact, these limitations apply to virtually any cognitive measure.

## TABLE 2-1

### Limitations of the WISC III

(1) The WISC III subtests measure learned information. In other words, it serves as an achievement test by assessing past accomplishments that are predictive of future academic success.

(2) The WISC III subtests are samples of behavior and not exhaustive. Therefore, the Full Scale IQ score should not be interpreted as an estimate of a child's global or total intellectual functioning.

(3) The WISC III assesses mental functioning under fixed experimental conditions.

(4) The WISC III is optimally useful when it is interpreted from an informational processing model. Taking from Luria's basic tenets, the model should include an input state, integration stage, storage capacity stage, and output stage.

(5) Hypotheses generated from the WISC III profile scores should be supported with data from multiple sources.

The *K-ABC* was designed to measure the cognitive processes underlying general intellectual functioning. It marked a radical departure from more traditional tests of intellectual functioning because of its reduced emphasis on verbal abilities and knowledge of specific content. Furthermore, the *K-ABC* played a significant role in the stagnant evolution of intelligence testing as it reinvigorated the notion of test development coinciding with actual theories of intelligence. The Mental Processing Composite (MPC) is based on two global subscales that assess a child's style of problem solving. The ability to process information in a serial order was termed the *Sequential Processing* subscale, while integrating several pieces of information at once as a whole or gestalt was called the *Simultaneous Processing* subscale. Though criticized for utilizing such ambiguous processing terms (sequential and simultaneous) as well as offering a simplistic brain-behavioral dichotomy of how information is processed (Sattler, 1988), the *K-ABC* stimulated a cognitive revolution among psychologists in the evaluation of higher cortical functions within the framework of multiple neurodevelopmental constructs. However, the popularity of the Wechsler-based framework of single numeric scores representing verbal and nonverbal abilities can still be seen in the advent of newer nonverbal assessments such as the *UNIT* and *TONI-3*.

Recently, the **Cognitive Assessment System (CAS)** was published by Naglieri (1997) and is based rather loosely on Luria's information processing model. The PASS theory, used as the theoretical basis for the CAS, viewed intelligence as a dynamic amalgamation of cognitive processes as opposed to a single, fixed, unitary measure. According to this theory, human cognitive functioning includes four primary components (Naglieri, 1999):

### TABLE 2-2

(1) *Planning* – the processes involved with cognitive control, utilization of processes and knowledges, intentionality, and self-regulation to achieve a desired goal.

(2) *Attention* – processes to provide focused and selective attention to an activity and resist distraction.

(3) *Simultaneous* – processing information into a single whole or group.

(4) *Successive* – processing information into a serial or temporal order.

Therefore, the attention subtests represent the first block or input stage of cognitive functioning, the simultaneous and successive subtests reflect the second block or perceptual integration stage of cognitive functioning, and the planning stage represents the output stage or third functional unit or block. An impressive feature of the *Cognitive Assessment System* remains its strong correlation (.70) with academic achievement measures, higher than any other intelligence test measure (Naglieri, 1999). Still, supporters of the factor analytic model of intelligence testing have levied criticism of this measure, claiming insufficient factorial support to justify the four PASS constructs (Carroll, 1995). Additionally, there are no formal language measures assessed given the author's notion of language representing a learned skill and ability and not necessarily reflecting a specific cognitive construct.

In summary, the evolution of intelligence testing remains in its infancy in capturing the cortical complexity and realm of possibilities which human cognitive functioning may take. Table 2-3 lists the current and most popular intelligence tests used by psychologists today, with the Wechsler series continuing to dominate the market. However, the past 100 years of measuring cortical functions have spawned various theories along the evolutionary path toward quantifying human cognition. Fueled in part by the technological advances of neuroimaging techniques, the disciplines of neurology, psychology, education, and medicine have begun to converge toward an amalgam or hybrid field known as neuropsychology. In fact, a neuropsychological paradigm can be a more powerful way of interpreting intelligence tests from a qualitative process-oriented approach. Therefore, a WISC-III supplemented by a WISC-III PI can be invaluable in understanding students error patterns. Refreshingly, the appreciation of individual variation during childhood has led researchers to explore the development and expression of the nearly 100 billion neurons and neuroglial cells that comprise the human brain. This staggering volume of neurons resonates louder when one considers that to count each neuron individually, one per second, it would take some 32 million years. Thus, neuropsychological research has focused on the neural networks and anatomical circuitry that make up various cognitive constructs such as attention, memory, language, processing speed, and graphomotor functioning. Similarly, Kaufman has stressed that intelligence testing should be interpreted within a conceptual model around given cognitive constructs (Kaufman, 1994), no matter what test is chosen. Therefore, the emphasis should not revolve around the measurement of *intelligence* per se, but rather on the measurement of *cognition*, which refers to the underlying constructs necessary to perform a given task.

## Table 2-3

### Intelligence Test Measures

| Name/publisher | IQ Ranges | Age Ranges | Testing Time | Definition & special features |
|---|---|---|---|---|
| Wechsler Intelligence Scale for Children – 3rd Ed. {WISC-III} 1991  *Psychological Corporation* | Verbal Scale: 46 –155 Performance Scale: 46-155 Full Scale: 40-160 | 6-16:11 yrs. | Core Subtests: 50-70 mins. | Measures children's intellectual ability according to Verbal Performance and Full Scale IQs. Also provides factor-based index scores for verbal comprehension, perceptual organization, freedom from distractibility, and processing speed. |
| Wechsler Primary & Preschool Scale of Intelligence – Revised {WPPSI-R}, 1989  *Psychological Corporation* | Verbal Scale: 46-160 Performance Scale: 45-160 Full Scale: 41-160 | 3-7:3 yrs. | 75 mins. | Clinical intelligence instrument developed for use with younger children. Has one group of primarily perceptual motor {performance} subtests and another of verbal subtests. Both groups yield IQs and, when combined, yield the full IQ. |
| Wechsler Adult Intelligence Scale – 3rd Ed. {WAIS-III}, 1997  *Psychological Corporation* | Verbal Scale: 48-155 Performance Scale: 47-155 Full Scale: 41-155 | 16-89 yrs. | 69-90 mins. | Generates IQ and index scores {with the exception of working memory for freedom from distractibility} similar to the WISC-III. |
| Kaufman Assessment Battery for Children {K-ABC}, 1983  *American Guidance Service* | Ages:     IQs 2:6-2:11  69-160 3:0-3:11  55-160 4:0-4:11  52-160 5:0-5:11  46-160 6:0-12:5  40-160 | 2:6-12:6 yrs. | 33-85 mins. | Assesses the intelligence and achievement levels of children. Generates global scaled scores for sequential, simultaneous, and mental processing. The achievement scale focuses on acquired facts and applied skills. |
| Kaufman Adult & Adolescent Intelligence Test {KAIT}, 1993  *Psychological Corporation* | Crystallized IQ: 40-160 Fluid IQ: 40-157 Composite IQ: 40-160 | 11-85+ yrs. | Core battery: 60 mins;  Expanded battery: 90 mins. | Test composed of crystallized and fluid scales of intelligence organized into a 6-subtest core battery and a 10-subtest expanded battery. Also offers a brief mental status test {supplementary}. Whether the core or expanded battery is given, the standard scores are based only on the 6 core subtests. |

| Name/publisher | IQ Ranges | Age Ranges | Testing Time | Definition & special features |
|---|---|---|---|---|
| Woodcock-Johnson, III {WJ-III} 2000<br><br>*Riverside Publishing* | Extended standard scores:<br><br>24-200 | 2-90+ yrs. | 5 mins. per subtest | Standard battery is comprised of 7 tests measuring verbal ability, thinking ability, and cognitive efficiency. There are 7 additional tests in the Extended battery in addition to 6 supplemental measures, yielding 20 cognitive tests in total. These tests are categorized by seven broad GF-GC factors of cognitive ability, based upon the Horn-Cattell & Carroll factor analytic model. |
| Stanford Binet – 4th Ed. {SB-4E}, 1986<br><br>*Riverside Publishing* | Each standard age score {SAS} and test composite; 36-164 | 2-23:11 yrs. | 33-85 mins. | Subtests each assess one of the following subject areas; verbal reasoning, quantitative reasoning, abstract/visual reasoning, and memory. Examinee is given a vocabulary test that serves as a routing test to determine the starting level for all other tests. |
| Cognitive Assessment System {CAS} 1997<br><br>*Riverside Publishing* | Planning Scale<br>Attention Scale<br>Simultaneous Scale<br>Successive Scale  40-160 | 5-17:11 yrs. | 40-60 mins. | Measure of intelligence based on the PASS Theory. Test assesses planning, attention, successive, and simultaneous processing. |
| British Abilities Scales {BAS II} 1996<br><br>NFER-Nelson {UK} | Preschool:<br>Gen'l. conceptual ability score {CGA}:<br>Age 2:6-3:5:  45-159<br>Age 3:6-5:11:  37-162<br>Verbal ability:  50-151<br>Nonverbal reasoning ability:  43-162<br>Spatial ability:  49-150<br>Special nonverbal composite {SNC}:<br>Age 2:6-3:5:  51-152<br>Age 3:6-5:11:  44-156 | Preschool:<br>2:6-5:11<br><br>School Age:<br>6:0-17:11 | 30-45 mins. | Yields a general conceptual ability {GCA} that denotes g, the general factor. All subtests contributing to the GCA are highly g loaded. For school-aged children, the BAS-II is formed from three clusters: Verbal, Nonverbal Reasoning, and Spatial. These clusters are interpretable as Gc {crystallized ability}, GF {fluid ability}, and Gv {broad visualization} in the Horn-Cattell & Carroll models. These three factors are the most highly correlated with higher-order g. Also provides a special nonverbal composite {SNC} which is a measure of g with the contribution of the verbal tests removed. |

| Name/publisher | IQ Ranges | Age Ranges | Testing Time | Definition & special features |
|---|---|---|---|---|
| British Abilities Scales {BAS II} 1996<br><br>*NFER-Nelson {UK}* | School age:<br>Gen'l. conceptual ability score {CGA}: 39-160<br>Verbal ability: 52-148<br>Nonverbal reasoning ability: 49-150<br>Spatial ability: 47-152<br>Special nonverbal composite {SNC}: 41-158 | | | |
| Differential Abilities Scales {DAS} 1990<br><br>*Psychological Corporation* | Preschool:<br>Gen'l. conceptual ability score {GCA}:<br>Age 2:6-3:5: 44-169<br>Age 3:6-5:11: 44-175<br>Verbal ability: 50-153<br>Nonverbal reasoning ability: 43-162<br>Spatial ability: 49-150<br>Special nonverbal composite {SNC}:<br>Age 2:6-3:5: 45-158<br>Age 3:6-5:11: 43-162<br><br>School Age:<br>Gen'l. conceptual ability score {GCA}: 45-164<br>Verbal ability: 51-151<br>Nonverbal reasoning ability: 52-152<br>Spatial ability: 50-155<br>Special nonverbal composite {SNC}: 48-162 | Preschool:<br>2:6-5:11 yrs.:<br><br>School Age:<br>6:0-17:11 yrs. | Full cognitive battery:<br>45-65 mins. | Consists of a cognitive battery of 17 subtests, divided into two overlapping age levels. Produces a general conceptual ability score composed of reasoning and conceptual abilities, a nonverbal composite, and cluster composite scores derived from the core subtests. |

| Name/publisher | IQ Ranges | Age Ranges | Testing Time | Definition & special features |
|---|---|---|---|---|
| Leiter International Performance Scale, 1948 <br> *Stoelting Company* | Adjusted IQ score: 25-160 | 2-28 yrs. | 30-45 mins. | Nonverbal test of intelligence used to evaluate children with sensory, motor, or language deficits. Contains 54 subtests. |
| Leiter International Performance Scale-Revised {Leiter-R}, 1997 <br> *Stoelting Company* | Brief IQ screener: 36-169 <br> Full Scale IQ: 30-170 | 2-2:11 yrs. | Varies | Used to evaluate cognitive functions, including measure of nonverbal intelligence, fluid reasoning, and visualization, visual-spatial memory, and attention. Very different structure and format from the previous version of the Leiter. |
| Universal Nonverbal Intelligence Test {UNIT}, 1998 <br> *Riverside Publishing* | Full Scale {abbreviated}: 45-153 <br> Full Scale {standard}: 41-159 <br> Full Scale {extended}: 40-159 | 5-17:11 yrs. | Abbreviated battery: 10-15 mins. <br> Standard battery: 30 mins. <br> Expanded battery: 40 mins. | Measure of children and adolescents who may be at a disadvantage in traditional verbal- and language-loaded tests. Although it is entirely nonverbal, it is designed to provide assessment of general intelligence, cognitive abilities, and memory. |
| Test of Nonverbal Intelligence-3 {TONI-3}, 1997 <br> *Pro-Ed* | Deviation quotient: 6_150 | 5-85+ yrs. | 15-20 mins. | Language-free measure that assesses intelligence, aptitude, abstract reasoning, and problem solving. Because no reading, writing, speaking, or listening is required, this test is often used with individuals whose language ability is limited or suspect. |
| Ravens: <br> {1} Colored Progressive Matrices; <br> {2} Standard Progressive Matrices: <br> {3} Advanced Progressive Matrices, 1986 <br> *Psychological Corporation* | Ranges vary, depending on age: 30-141 | {1} 5-11:11 yrs., physically impaired; <br> {2} 6-16 yrs., 18+ yrs.; <br> {3} 12-16 yrs., 18+ yrs. | 20-45 mins. <br> 20-45 mins. <br> 40-60 mins. | Nonverbal test of reasoning ability presented in three different forms. Can be administered individually or to a group. Scores are converted into percentile ranks. |

Perhaps no other academic task requires the unique synchronization and harmony of multiple cognitive constructs performing at peak efficiency more than written language. Obviously, a strong linguistic base is required, though the sequential ordering of words on paper, the graphomotor execution of the hand manipulating a pencil, the ability to focus and sustain attention skills, the efficacy of word retrieval strategies, and the necessary planning and organizational skills all contribute to this sophisticated linguistic endeavor. If children cannot express themselves in written form, it impacts on their learning ability in every subject area. Writing skills must be emphasized in kindergarten and continually reinforced throughout a child's academic career. As a process generated internally and expressed externally on paper, written language may be conceptualized as the reverse of neuropsychological process of reading. Hence, writing starts as a perception of an external stimulus and is subsequently processed internally. There is no doubt that school success hinges on the appropriate development of skills in reading and writing - therefore it is crucial for educators to understand the fundamental psychological processes that contribute to each. In essence, written language represents the pinnacle of higher cognitive functioning as multiple lexical and perceptual processes are required to perform this task. Furthermore, breakdowns in one or multiple processes can contribute to various elements of **dysgraphia**, which is a disorder of written expression. Table 2-4 lists the essential neurodevelopmental constructs and their subsequent contribution to the writing process.

## TABLE 2—4

| NEURODEVELOPMENTAL CONSTRUCT | POSSIBLE IMPACTS ON WRITTEN LANGUAGE |
|---|---|
| Attention | • Poor planning<br>• Uneven tempo<br>• Erratic legibility<br>• Inconsistent spelling & use of conventions<br>• Uneven memory flow<br>• Poor self-monitoring, careless errors<br>• Lack of persistence |
| Spatial Production | • Poor spatial planning of page<br>• Deficient visualization of words & letters<br>• Poor margination<br>• Organization problems<br>• Deficient {dyseidetic} spelling<br>• Uneven spacing between letters & words<br>• Poor use of lines |
| Sequential Production | • Slow learning of serial motor movements for letter forms & connected writing<br>• Letter transpositions & omissions in spelling<br>• Poor narrative sequencing<br>• Organization problems<br>• Lack of transitions & cohesive ties |
| Memory | • Weak word retrieval<br>• Deficient spelling<br>• Fluctuating recall of motor engrams for letters<br>• Poor recall of rules {inadequate application of punctuation, capitalization, grammar}<br>• Dysfluent writing<br>• Poor legibility<br>• Preference for printing over cursive writing<br>• Loss of train of thought |

| NEURODEVELOPMENTAL CONSTRUCT | POSSIBLE IMPACTS ON WRITTEN LANGUAGE |
|---|---|
| Language | • Impoverished vocabulary<br>• Poor written expression<br>• Dysphonetic spelling<br>• Vague referencing<br>• Lack of cohesive ties<br>• Awkward phrasing & unconventional grammar<br>• Inappropriate use of colloquial language<br>• Inadequate narration<br>• Simplistic sentence structures & lack of variety |
| High-order Cognition | • Constricted, simplistic, concrete ideation<br>• Lack of development of ideas & descriptive elaboration<br>• Poor audience awareness<br>• Paucity of written output<br>• Weak opinion development |
| Graphomotor | • Diminished amount of writing<br>• Slow writing<br>• Effort writing {sometimes "eclipsing" other functions}<br>• Poor legibility<br>• Awkward pencil grip<br>• Lack of fluidity in cursive writing<br>• Preference for printing |

*Adapted from Levine, M.D., & Reed, M., (1999). *Developmental Variation and Learning Disorders.* Massachusetts: Educators Publishing Service, Inc.

# fostering Motivation in Developing writers

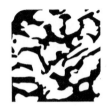

## Chapter 3

"The pen is mightier than the sword."
— Anonymous

Most professional sports organizations spend millions of dollars in the highly mercurial market of player development, or what used to be called scouting. The success or failure of a given franchise in the multi-billion-dollar sports entertainment industry often hinges on their efficiency in evaluating human athletic prowess for a specific endeavor. Scores of professionals spend countless hours reviewing videotapes of past performances, while scouting combines, super-camps, and individual workout sessions provide more personal glimpses of potential players. As teams become more interested in specific athletes, psychological profiles are mandated, educational histories are sought, and invasive background checks rivaling those of the CIA are undertaken prior to selecting an individual player. Since most team sports such as football and basketball rely heavily on speed and strength, quantitative measures are often employed to statistically categorize would-be players seeking to make their fortunes in what is essentially a child's game. For instance, specific measures such as lateral speed, vertical jumping ability, 40-yard dash time, and the ability to bench-press weights exceeding 225 pounds are filed and catalogued for each athlete.

Still, the vast majority of players who succeed on a professional level are generally overlooked by most scouting departments, while many athletes who were highly successful in college fail miserably on the professional level. In other words, despite the efforts of professional scouting departments to select the most likely candidates carefully for their respective sports organizations, most marquee players on a professional level tend to blossom unexpectedly. For instance, among the top eight quarterbacks in the National Football League, none were selected in the first round of the draft by their respective teams, but they nevertheless emerged as elite performers through hard work, dedication, and perseverance. One could argue quite convincingly that attempting to quantify athletic prowess for predictive purposes, namely deciphering who might be most successful on the professional level, is more art than science. However, temperament characteristics such as intrinsic motivation, persistence, emotional resiliency, and ability to cope with pressure are perhaps variables and traits more determinant of being a successful athlete than times in the 40-yard dash.

Attempting to quantify a student's written language capabilities in an overly mechanistic way can also be extremely misleading. Most educators and diagnosticians should take note of the aforementioned sports analogy when attempting to determine who might be a successful writer versus who might be at risk for academic failure. Simply put, the same temperamental attributes leading to success on the athletic field may also be a better predictor of success in the classroom than simply relying on rote statistical measures such as quantifying intelligence through IQ test scores. After all, intelligence test scores do not measure important attributes for learning such as motivation, creativity, flexibility of thought, or personality styles. Therefore, motivation and desire to succeed may be the most crucial elements for success in virtually any academic endeavor, especially written language.

A growing body of evidence suggests that highly motivated writers are able to use a variety of approaches and strategies that are dependent on their purposes and audiences. Boice (1994) contended that most capable writers recognize that written expression is a way of entering a kind of conversation leading to self-understanding and interaction with others. Skilled writers tend to hold positive views about the utility of writing, engaging in their task with anticipation, feelings of control, and minimal anxiety. Their writing production is steady and relatively stress-free. Unfortunately, many people do not experience their writing development with such ease. For instance, according to the National Center for Education Statistics (1997), writing assessment indicated that while 80% of eleventh graders can indeed write focused and clear responses to assignments, fewer than one-third can write complete responses containing information to support their claims. Alarmingly, only 2% can write effective responses that contain supporting details and discussion.

It is important to note that in addition to teaching the mechanics of composition, there is evidence of significant failure to develop students' positive beliefs and motivation towards writing. Boice (1994) observed that students who experienced a limited amount of written language success often *force writing with a hurried pace, a lagging confidence, and a lingering malaise*. Furthermore, these students remain ambivalent about writing and inconsistent about turning intentions into actions. Although many students acknowledge that writing is important and directly related to success in school and life, the thought of writing too often evokes reactions that are negative, such as feelings of anxiety and dread, lack of control, and avoidance (Cleary, 1991).

In spite of the need to learn about fostering the motivation to write, there is solid theory and research about the processes of writing itself. Much of this scholarship was conducted in the past twenty years. In both the cognitive sciences and the literary tradition, studies report that writing is a process of *meaning making*. Skilled writing is now acknowledged for what it is: a very complex problem-solving act that involves memory, planning, text generation, and revision (Flower et. al., 1990). Writers must switch attention between multiple goals (Hayes, 1996) and satisfy numerous constraints of topic, audience, purpose, and of physically creating the text itself. In fact, the ability to switch back and forth among numerous frames of reference such as critical thinking skills, rhetorical stances, and writing conventions is a hallmark feature of executive functioning skills (see Chapter 7). In a task as complex and difficult as writing, motivational issues assume prominent status. Writers need to develop strong beliefs in the relevance and importance of writing as they grapple with its complexities and frustrations and learn the virtues of patience, persistence and flexibility. These beliefs about writing ability do fall within the realm of intrinsic motivation, but it is also true that the development of motivation for writing is largely the responsibility of those who set the writing tasks and react to what has been written - namely, parents and educators.

Most researchers investigating motivational aspects of writing, such as Bruning and Horn (2000), have argued for an expansion of writing models to more explicitly recognize the social and cognitive variables implicit in the literature. Literacy research has long emphasized the need to help students learn not only how to write, but also how to want to write (Spaulding 1992). A vast body of research has addressed issues of student interest, engagement, and motivation. However, as Spaulding (1992) noted, most of these studies have not been examined with respect to specific studies of writing. The wealth of knowledge on practical instruction about writing is informative, but there remains a lack of scientific analysis aimed at the critical factors of writing motivation.

A general framework for research aimed at understanding written language development develops from several basic assumptions. The first assumption argues that the root source of motivation to write stems from a core set of beliefs about the writing process. Motivational considerations are an essential aspect of a writer's self-conception, given that writers must make trade-offs between the costs and benefits of various goals and strategies when writing (Flower et al., 1990). In any written language endeavor, writers must negotiate between what is expected and what can be realistically done. This is a challenging task and students need to be sufficiently motivated to enter, persist, and succeed in this complicated problem space known as writing.

A second assumption is that the source of motivation is experiencing writing as a purposeful and authentic form of communication (Crystal, 1997). Written expression must be conceived of not so much as a product, but also a process and a way of entering and participating in discourse (Boice, 1994). The central guiding force underlying this conception is the teacher, whose conceptions of writing often provide a model for shaping a student's belief and molding their self-confidence. Thus, programs for developing written language motivation must rest on the core values and beliefs held by teachers themselves.

A third assumption is that understanding the motivation to write demands an appreciation of the relationship between writing and oral language. Many of the conditions that support the phenomenon of oral language acquisition can also be applied to written expression. The difference between oral and written communication must be understood, and writing development cannot be accomplished simply by creating a literacy-rich environment. Table 3-1 contrasts the features of written and oral discourse. Obviously, writing is a more deliberate and formal act than speech. Learning to write is a very complex linguistic and cognitive task that requires close attention to the conditions for developing both motivation and skill. Since written language tends to be removed from experience, it often lacks the type of context that supports oral discourse. The unique challenge for the writer is to recreate a lived or imagined experience without the immediacy of oration (Cameron et. al., 1996). Learning to read may be facilitated by oral language experiences, with parents encouraging understanding by speaking in literary ways, but writing also needs the same type of support structure. Written discourse contains many unfamiliar elements and exposes a writer's thoughts and feelings to far greater scrutiny. Careful planning is required to develop motivation for writing. As Bruning and Horn (2000) conclude, the motivational challenge for a teacher involves reassuring students that the benefits of effortful writing far outweigh its considerable risks. The most critical conditions in developing writing motivation suggested by these authors are outlined in Table 3-2.

## TABLE 3-1

### Typical features of children's experience with oral and written discourse

**Oral Discourse**

- Rapid, transitory, inexact, variable. The provision of additional information is a major
- Mechanism for refining meanings and correcting errors.
- Contextual and implicit. Listeners can "fill in" meaning using a variety of contextual clues.
- Early, high, continuing exposure. Most children are immersed in rich discourse communities that link oral language to all parts of their lives.
- Highly varied pragmatic uses. Most beginning students are skilled at using natural language to describe things, tell stories, and express their feelings.
- Narrative structures dominate. Communication success depends on imagery, memorability, and implicit meanings.

**Written Discourse**

- Slow developing, stable, and reproduceable. Revision in light of communication purpose and audience is critical for clarifying ideas and communicating effectively.
- Decontextualized and explicit. Writers must establish common ground for understanding, considering factors such as purpose, audience, and writing conventions.
- Later, lower, more intermittent exposure. Most children entering school are relative novices at writing, unsure about writing's uses and their own capabilities.
- Narrower range of uses. Most entering students will not yet have used writing pragmatically and need to discover writing's utility for description, self-expression, and persuasion.
- Descriptive, logical structures dominate. Writing permits careful examination of cognitive and emotional dimensions of communication. Successful writing requires mastery of formal language conventions.

## TABLE 3-2

### Factors in Developing Motivation to Write

**Nurturing functional beliefs about writing**

- Creating a classroom community supporting writing and other literacy activities.
- Displaying the ways that teachers use writing personally.
- Finding writing tasks that assure student success.
- Providing opportunities for students to build expertise in areas they will write about.
- Using brief daily writing activities to encourage regular writing.
- Encouraging writing in a wide variety of genres.

**Fostering student engagement through authentic writing goals and contexts**

- Having students find examples of different kinds of writing (e.g. self-expressive, persuasive, entertaining).
- Encouraging students to write about topics of personal interest.
- Having students write for a variety of audiences.
- Establishing improved communication as purpose for revision.
- Integrating writing into instruction in other disciplines (e.g. science, math, social studies).

**Providing a supportive context for writing**

- Breaking complex writing tasks into parts.
- Encouraging goal setting and monitoring of progress.
- Assisting students in setting writing goals that are neither too challenging nor too simple.
- Teaching writing strategies and helping students learn to monitor their use.
- Giving feedback on progress toward writing goal.
- Using peers as writing partners in literacy communities.

**Creating a positive emotional environment**

- Modeling positive attitudes towards writing.
- Creating a safe environment for writing.
- Giving students choices about what they will write.
- Providing feedback allowing students to retain control over their writings.
- Utilizing natural outcomes (e.g., communication success) as feedback source.
- Training students to engage in positive self-talk about writing.
- Helping students reframe anxiety, stress as natural arousal.

*Adapted from Bruning and Horn (2000). Developing motivation to write, *Educational Psychologist*, 35(1), 25-37.

Writing is a complex task, and success in this endeavor requires engagement in extended periods of concentration. Cognitive, linguistic, and motivational resources are all utilized in the process. To sustain concentration throughout the difficult and emotional process of writing, students must have a healthy self-conception of their potential for written expression. The primary belief, according to Codling & Gambrell (1997), must be that writing has an inherent value. Most students acknowledge that it does, especially for achieving academic success and career goals. What must follow then is developing a sense of competence as a writer. This assumption is supported by the recurrence of the self-efficacy theory in literature on writing motivation. Writing skill and efficacy have been linked to show that high efficacy writers demonstrate lower anxiety, greater persistence, and higher toleration for frustration in writing tasks (Bruning & Horn, 2000).

Like most theoretical models, written language appears to follow a rather prescriptive developmental course. In fact, most neurolinguistic communication abilities tend to develop in a rather fixed sequence of receptive and expressive skills, with oral language being the foundation both for reading and written language. The ability to expand and utilize our vocabulary helps us to organize our thoughts in speech, and is a necessary prerequisite for efficient reading and writing skills. When younger children develop deficits in oral expression, the foundation for enhancing more sophisticated communication skills, specifically written communication, becomes compromised. Writing subskills that need to be specifically targeted include handwriting, spelling, grammar, and syntax. The writing process entails adequate planning and organizational skills that need to be drafted, corrected, rewritten, and revised. Educators need to reinforce and model effective written language, almost as an emerging work of art that needs to be refined and modified constantly to be perfected. All proficient writers have an ebb and flow to their ideas that convey intent, capture emotion, and sequentially unfold a level of thought. Teaching text structure and helping children use strategies to write fluently will ensure success and lead to more positive self-conceptions.

Therefore, it could be argued that positive self-conceptions stem from the result of improvements in written language competence. For example, compared to fourth-graders, both seventh and tenth graders were found to have higher self-efficacy for completing writing tasks (Shell et. al., 1995). Some researchers (Schunk & Swartz, 1993) have demonstrated that self-efficacy for writing is also linked to the specific strategies being deployed by students, in addition to the encouragement and positive feedback received. In fact, students with learning disabilities who were taught strategies for composition writing improved both their writing skills and self-efficacy. Moreover, these improvements were transferred to other learning tasks. Schunk and Swartz (1993) found that elementary students who were taught about writing process goals and given progress feedback demonstrated progress in self-efficacy, especially when the interventions were used in tandem. In summary, most interventions have the greatest chance for success when they convey a belief to students that they are indeed capable of continued writing improvement. This belief can then inspire continued motivation, effort, and resiliency to become more proficient writers.

It is important to note that positive motivational consequences which foster environments that provide students an opportunity for input and choice, promote student interaction, and provide challenging tasks tend to be most successful. These considerations are particularly useful when encouraging lower ability writers. Meece and Miller (1993) reported that students find cognitively complex learning activities inherently more interesting and demanding of mental efforts. Furthermore, Turner (1995) argued that such tasks lead to higher levels of motivation because they create interest, allow for self-improvement, and afford opportunities to control one's own learning. Writers need to believe, however, that complex tasks can be accomplished with reasonable effort. Such a belief can be fostered when writing tasks are defined for students with clear goals and standards for success.

Since most written language opportunities are presented in school, teachers are largely responsible for choosing appropriate assignments and interventions that hopefully will bolster motivation. In addition to providing guidance and feedback on writing assignments, teachers can best help developing writers by breaking writing tasks into manageable parts. This not only reduces the processing demands of writing, but it also allows time for students to self-monitor their progress during the writing process. Hence, each writing task serves to reinforce a student's beliefs about their writing ability, the amount of time they are willing to invest in the assignment, and about the value of their success.

Lastly, developing motivation to write is often dependent on the creation of a positive emotional environment. Hayes and Daiker (1984) found that the single most important factor in a writing environment was positive reinforcement. Teachers should offer praise with the same intensity as they point out mistakes. A safe environment where ideas are treated with respect will also encourage students to express themselves with openness. Where there is an atmosphere of trust, caring, and mutual concern, students are motivated to engage in the writing process. As stated previously, writers must feel that they have some measure of control over their writing task.

Successful writing experiences most often occur when students have working knowledge of the topic. Motivation, interest, organization and belief in the value of writing are likely to result from writing assignments on topics on which students have content mastery. Writing-strategy training can also lessen the sheer anxiety that most students feel once task demands increase. Breaking writing assignments into sections and receiving feedback on progress toward writing goals can facilitate and help foster motivation to write.

# subtypes of Language-based Dysgraphias

## Chapter 4

*"It's a damn poor mind that can only think of one way to spell a word."*
— *Andrew Johnson*

The current nomenclature for the identification of a specific written language impairment is rather imprecise and relatively ill-conceived, leaving diagnosticians, educators, and parents grappling for further explanations and direction. Consider the diagnostic criteria for disorders of written expression as listed by the Diagnostic and Statistical Manual of Mental Disorders: Fourth Edition (DSM IV):

---

### Diagnostic criteria for 315.2 Disorder of Written Expression

A.  Writing skills, as measured by individually administered standardized tests or functional assessments of writing skills, are substantially below those expected given the person's chronological age, measured intelligence, and age-appropriate education.
B.  The disturbance in Criterion A significantly interferes with academic achievement or activities of daily living that require the composition of written texts (e.g. writing grammatically correct sentences and organized paragraphs).
C.  If a sensory deficit is present, the difficulties in writing skills are in excess of those usually associated with it.

---

*Diagnostic and Statistical Manual of Mental Disorders: Fourth Edition (1994). American Psychiatric Association: Washington DC.

There are a number of faults inherent within this set of criteria. First, no psychometric guidelines are given that reflect how extensively a student must be working below age, grade, or intelligence levels before a disability is truly manifested. Second, no developmental guidelines are mentioned, and therefore the same criteria used to judge a 1st grader's penmanship skills would be applied toward evaluating a 12th grade student's expository writing capabilities. Third, the vague terminology "significantly interferes with academic achievement" needs to be clarified and operationally defined. Fourth, the set of criteria is extraordinarily simplistic, indicating that a disability persists merely if a student performs poorly in a particular skill. Thus, if William Shakespeare suffered a debilitating head injury with significant frontal lobe impairment, thus rendering him incapable of composing prosaic masterpieces though still able to draft a letter, would he necessarily be impaired?

Unfortunately, most school systems, educational practices, and clinical settings use some form of discrepancy between academic achievement and purported level of general intelligence to determine the presence of a disability. In fact, since its passage in 1975, perhaps no other documentation or single piece of legislation has more profoundly impacted the nature of determining learning handicaps than Public Law 94-142, the Education for All Handicapped Children Act. With respect to a specific learning disability, most educational institutions adhere to the following criteria:

*Specific learning disability means a disorder in one or more of the basic psychological processes involved in understanding or in using language, spoken or written, which may manifest itself in an imperfect ability to listen, think, speak, read, write, spell, or perform mathematical calculations. The term includes such conditions as perceptual handicaps, brain injury, minimal brain dysfunction, dyslexia and developmental aphasia. The term does not include children who have learning problems which are primarily the result of visual, hearing or motor handicaps, of mental retardation, of emotional disturbance, or of environmental, cultural, or economic disadvantage. (Sattler, p.598)*

Though more comprehensive than the DSM IV criterion, especially with respect to differential diagnosis, Public Law 94-142 simply relies on a discrepancy between academic performance and intellectual functioning to determine the presence of an educational disability. Despite being amended in 1997 under the Individuals with Disabilities Educational Act (IDEA), the law still insists that a diagnosis of "*specific learning disability*" should be applied only to children with a significant discrepancy between academic achievement and intellectual ability in one or more receptive skills, such as written expression, listening and reading comprehension, and/or mathematics.

As mentioned previously, numerous pitfalls exist in relying on a *discrepancy model* for the assessment of a specific learning disorder, some of which include the tendency to preclude early identification due to psychometric limitations, poor developmental sensitivity, and lack of agreement on measurement criterion (Feifer & DeFina, 2000). Notwithstanding, Chapter 2 highlighted the limitations of intelligence testing and the poor distinction between the knowledge, skills, and abilities that comprise intellectual functioning versus those that constitute academic achievement. As Kaufman (1994) succinctly pointed out, intelligence tests such as the WISC-III measure learned skills and past accomplishments predictive of educational success; therefore they really represent yet another measure of student achievement. Given the multiple perceptual and lexical processes involved in written expression, an entire paradigm shift toward a more sophisticated view of human cognitive functioning – or at least a more appropriate methodology - seems essential.

Written expression remains the final frontier in the evolution of human communication, emerging after comprehension, speech, and then reading (Sandler et. al, 1992). It is without question the highest form of language communication and therefore the most difficult to develop. The neuropsychological evaluation of linguistic functioning focuses on brain-behavioral relationships involved in the acquisition and utilization of language for a given skill. Since written language remains a relatively new skill according to evolutionary time tables, having only emerged in the past 5000 years, there is no one particular brain region yet to be designated or assigned to written production (Carter, 1998). Therefore, producing written language requires multiple linguistic skills involving phonological and orthographical functioning (the elementary components of language), the lexical level of functioning (semantics), syntax, and finally the level of discourse or pragmatics (Kertesz, 1994).

In order to evaluate these linguistic components properly, Luria created a process-oriented approach to assessment based on his disdain for fixed, psychometrically standardized batteries. Consequently, most practitioners in neuropsychology favor selecting individual subtests from a variety of batteries to measure specific constructs, and explore patterns of neurodevelopmental strengths and weaknesses based upon the areas in question. Whereas reading begins with visual stimuli in the outside environment and ends with the brain determining meaning from the stimuli, writing begins with an idea and intent to communicate within the brain, and ends with a psychomotor act that leaves a tangible record (Gaddes & Edgell, 1994). Hence, they are almost reverse neuropsychological processes. With respect to written language disorders, the following classification system should be helpful in assisting educators and diagnosticians toward pinpointing specific breakdowns in the written language process, and most importantly, implementing effective remediation techniques.

## TABLE 4–1

| classification of Dysgraphia | | | | | | | |
|---|---|---|---|---|---|---|---|
| Type | | Definition | Dictation and writing names of objects or actions | Can copy written words | Can copy mirror writing | Can copy diagrams | Mirror writing to dictation |
| Aphasic agraphia (language disorder) | Phonological | Cannot convert phoneme into grapheme | Phonologically incorrect misspellings | Yes | Yes | Yes | Yes |
| | Lexical (Surface) | Cannot learn or recall lexically (recognize whole word) | Phonologically correct misspellings | Yes | Yes | Yes | No |
| | Dyslexic (Mixed) | Cannot convert grapheme into grapheme with strephosymbolia and graphical (lexical) errors | Misspellings with reversals, omissions inversions and substitutions, non-words, and paragraphic errors | | Poor | Yes | No |
| | Gerstmann | Fluent incomprehensive order of letters and words | Misspellings with jumbled sentences | | Poor | Yes | No |
| | Semantic | Retarded or aphasic subjects | Generally below average performance | | Untidy | Untidy | Untidy |
| | Motor apraxic | Poor penmanship, as with clumsy child | Untidy with mild reversals; no paragraphia | | Yes | Yes | Yes |
| Apraxic agraphia (non-language disorder) | Ideational apraxic | Can copy; mild difficulty with dictation; cannot write names of objects or actions; cannot write spontaneously | Fair to poor | Yes | Poor | Poor | No |
| | Constructional apraxic | Visuospatial difficulty; cannot copy | Reversals and inversions; no paragraphia; untidy | | | | |
| Mechanical agraphia | | No cognitive dysfunction; mechanical problems with hands | Untidy | | Untidy | Untidy | Untidy |

*Adapted from Gubbay, S.S., & de Klerk, N.H., (1995). A study and review of developmental dysgraphia in relation to acquired dysgraphia. *Brain and Development*, 17, 1-8.

**Phonological Dysgraphia**: Phonological dysgraphia is a written language deficit characterized by writing and spelling disturbances in which the spelling of unfamiliar words, non-words, and phonetically irregular words is impaired. However, little impairment exists in a student's ability to copy words, write from dictation, or spell relatively familiar words. At the core of phonological dysgraphia is the inability to convert graphemes to phonemes, coupled with an inability to hold phonemes in memory and blend them in their appropriate sequence to produce the target word (Conway, et. al., 1998). In other words, a student experiences extreme difficulty manipulating the sound structure of spoken language, an essential component of the internal representation of words in print.

*Phonological awareness*, a blanket term often used in education, refers to higher-level linguistic tasks and a metacognitive understanding that spoken language is comprised of a series of sounds that occupy a particular sequential order. This differs from phonics knowledge, a lower-level paired-associate form of learning that relates letters and sounds on an automatic or rote level (Clark & Uhry, 1995). The hallmark feature of phonological dysgraphia lies in the inability to spell by sound, thus creating an over-reliance on the visual features of letters and words to assist with spelling. These students often memorize words in a rote or concrete manner based in large part on the unique visual contour or shape of a given word. With enough effort, these students may pass weekly spelling tests, though they often bewilder their teachers with their inability to spell the exact same word the following week or in a different context. Simply put, the brain is not organized to use solely visual pattern cues to memorize the multitude of configurations in which 26 letters can be arranged to represent some 80,000 words in the average lexicon. Consequently, the alphabetic code has emerged as a more viable mechanism to track the subtle nuances language may take through the vast simplification, deletion, and substitutions of phonemes and syllables in words. Interestingly, there appears to be evidence that certain categories of words such as nouns and adjectives are spelled better than verbs or function words (Baxter & Warrington, 1985). Nevertheless, the inability to spell pseudowords is the benchmark of this disorder (Alexander, et. al., 1992). Table 4-2 lists some common misspellings for dysphonetic spelling.

## TABLE 4-2

| Dysphonetic spelling errors | | |
| --- | --- | --- |
| Target word | Misspelling | Analysis |
| point | pot | phoneme substitution |
| train | chan | phoneme substitution |
| old | od | phoneme deletion |
| climbing | cling | phoneme deletion |
| job | joib | vowel substitution |
| video | veio | consonant omission |
| kitchen | tihn | consonant omission |

**Neuropsychological Significance:**  A behavior is the final common pathway by which learning is expressed, and is dependent on intact neural wiring in the brain coupled with adequate environmental experience and practice (Ohare & Brown, 1989). Therefore, dysphonetic spelling, when examined within a neuropsychological paradigm, is the observable by-product of faulty neurological pathways that subserve the spelling process. However, there remains some debate as to which regions are at fault. The evolution of the cerebral cortex has yielded certain brain regions primarily responsible for all language - oral, written, spoken, or reading. For 99 percent of right-handers and nearly 70 percent of left-handers, there is a left hemispheric dominance for language housed within the left temporal lobes (Kolb & Whishaw, 1996). Just as the visual system breaks down a specific visual image by color, form, and motion, with each being processed by a specialized region of the cortex, the language system is also subdivided and processed within various cortical regions (Calvin & Ojeman, 1994). The *superior temporal gyrus*, located on the uppermost crest of the temporal lobes, is critical for deciphering the 44 phonemes which comprise the English language. This is essentially where grapheme/phoneme analysis takes place, and thus remains a critical brain region for lower-level phonics knowledge. However, neuroimaging studies have suggested that the anterior portion of the *supramarginal gyrus* is the main culprit for disorders of phonological dysgraphia (Alexander et. al., 1992, Gubbay & deKlerk, 1995).

To appreciate the functional utility and heightened sophistication of this brain region, Goldberg's (1989) gradiential model of brain functioning offers amazing insight into the neural architecture of cerebral functioning. According to Goldberg (1989), the left temporal lobe involves categorical representation of auditory stimulus patterns. This function is critical for deciphering sound patterns that constitute words and language, as well as for the categorical perception of non-language sounds, such as a dog barking or a car backfiring. In many ways the concept of categorical processing of auditory perception can be viewed as the evolutionary and cultural precursor of language. The neuroanatomical location of the **supramarginal gyrus** lies at the intersection of the temporal and parietal lobes. The gradiental approach to brain functioning stipulates that any two brain regions or structures that are spatially close together in the brain have similar functional properties mediated between them. Therefore, the **supramarginal gyrus** functions to integrate the categorical representations of sounds (temporal lobe) with the spatial appreciation of sounds and symbols (inferior parietal lobe), and therefore plays a vital role in the spatial ordering of acoustical information. Should damage to this region occur, the net result is dysphonetic spelling characterized by the systematic simplification, deletion, and substitutions of phonemes and syllables in words, and the subsequent over-reliance on the visual features or orthography of words when spelling.

Many teachers have often commented that boys seem to have much more difficulty than girls on weekly spelling tests and in their overall written expression. With the prevalence of males to females in special education at approximately a 3:1 ratio, the prevailing attitude among most educators remains that writing and spelling skills are primarily effort-based skills. Hence, when academically challenged, boys tend to display greater outward signs of frustration, put forth minimal effort, and display an indifferent attitude toward more challenging academic endeavors given their more aggressive make-up. These stereotypical belief patterns unfortunately reflect 'pop' psychology's influence on the American psyche, claiming that girls outperform boys on linguistic tasks while boys outperform girls on more masculine endeavors such as spatial and mathematic skills. Perhaps the reason for this trend lies in the cytoarchitectural properties of the brain rather than the frivolous biases and trite overgeneralizations cited to explain learning differences between boys and girls. As can be seen by Figure 4-1, there appears to be more bilateral representation for phonological processing in the female brain. Therefore, a more plausible explanation for the overrepresentation of males in special education may include discussion of the multiple phonological processing sites of females which render back-up brain regions capable of modulating this function when needed. In contrast, the male brain exhibits more unilateral representation of phonological processing, namely in the left hemisphere, thus leaving itself more vulnerable to potential dysfunction since few other regions seem capable of subserving this skill. Perhaps the fact that the female brain tends to have **bilateral** representation for phonological processing explains why females are less likely than males to have significant decrements in their language skills following a left-hemispheric stroke (Shaywitz, 1996). As mentioned previously, there has been some debate regarding the exact anatomical location of dysphonetic dysgraphia, with some cases noting multiple lesion sites in addition to the supramarginal gyrus (Alexander et. al., 1992). Once again, some of the findings may reflect the subtle differences in the organizational properties between the male and female brain.

## fIGURE 4-1

### Brain Activation During phonological processing

Male Brain - unilateral processing          female Brain - bilateral processing

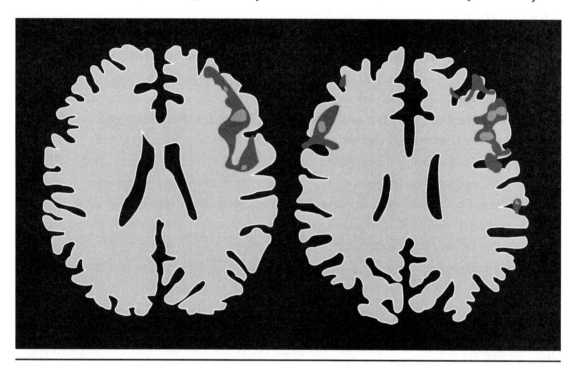

*Adapted from Lyon, G.R. & Rumsey, J.M. (1996). *Neuroimaging: A window to the neurological foundations of learning and behavior in children.* Baltimore: Paul H. Brookes Publishing Company. Printed with permission.

**Surface Dysgraphia:** Whereas phonological dysgraphia reflects a fundamental breakdown in the ability to spell due to difficulty segmenting words into their corresponding sequence of phonemes, *surface dysgraphia* reflects little difficulty with phoneme to grapheme conversion rules. Instead, this disorder is characterized by poor knowledge of the idiosyncratic properties of words, that is, poor lexical representations (Romani et. al., 1999). In other words, these children have little difficulty spelling by sound and appear capable of spelling non-words, though they struggle with phonetically irregular words containing alternative spelling patterns. Since most spelling miscues appear phonologically consistent, the hallmark feature of surface dysgraphia appears to be a breakdown in the orthographic representation of words, thereby causing the student to over-rely on sound patterns when spelling. Table 4-3 depicts typical spelling errors associated with surface dysgraphia.

TABLE 4-3

| surface dysgraphia spelling errors | |
|---|---|
| Target word | Misspelling |
| knock | nok |
| build | bild |
| mighty | mite |
| juice | juse |
| plate | plat |
| onion | unnyun |
| said | sed |
| yacht | yot |
| laugh | laf |

According to Frith & Frith (1983), the initial stages of reading and written language commence with a logographic phase in which children identify words on the basis of some distinctive visual feature, without necessarily recognizing all of the letters in their correct serial position. Next, children enter an alphabetic stage in which they learn the relationships between individual written letters and their corresponding sounds (phonemic awareness). Lastly, as children become more proficient in their reading and written language skills, they re-enter an orthographic stage in which words can be recognized and spelled correctly on the basis of their lexical or orthographic properties. In other words, skilled readers do not read familiar words in a sound-by-sound fashion but rather scan words based upon certain visual characteristics, thus allowing them to read in a fluent and automatic manner. Therefore, surface dysgraphics as well as surface dyslexics may have difficulty making the transition from the alphabetic stage of linguistic development to the orthographic processing stage. Table 4-4 illustrates the various stages of spelling development.

## TABLE 4-4

| stages in spelling development | | |
|---|---|---|
| spelling stage | Description | examples |
| Precommunicative | Knows some letter names and recognizes some printed letters, but does not understand correspondences between specific letters and sounds | *bqx* for *man*; *qit* for *order* |
| Semiphonetic | Realizes that letters represent speech sounds. Abbreviated spellings are used, primarily consonants. Single letters often are used to represent a whole word or syllable, and beginning and ending consonants are emphasized. | *lo* for *yellow*; *r* for *are*; *u* for *you*; *hs* for *house*; *misf* for *myself* |
| Phonetic | Learns to represent all phonemes in a word, using knowledge of letter names and letter-sound correspondences. Spelling patterns are heavily influenced by articulatory features of phonemes and remain simplified. The *ch* sound may be represented by *h*, and the *sh* sound by *h* or *s*. The *y* sound, as in *yellow* may be represented by *u*, and the *w* sound, as in *water*, may be represented by *y*. Long vowel sounds are represented by single letters. Short vowel sounds are represented by letters articulated in the same position. | *gen* for *green*; *at* for *eight*; *yit* for *wet*; *sak* for *shake*; *sreg* for *spring*; *pat* for *plant*; *huy* for *who*; *fes* for *fish*; *jes* for *dress*; *chk* or *chuk* for *truck*; *hk* for *chick*; *segeg* for *singing*; *haheg* for *hatching*; *masl* for *muscle* |
| Transitional | Child learns that most sounds are represented by more than one letter. Becomes aware of silent letters, double vowel patterns, double consonants, and common syllable patterns. Child may overgeneralize or undergeneralize rules and mis-sequence letters while practicing with more advanced spelling concepts. Spellings may become less accurate phonemically during this transitional phase. | *hase* for *house*; *appoole* for *apple*; *tallist* for *tallest*; *cou* for *cow*; *light* for *light*; *cach* for *catch*; *maek* for *make* |

*Adapted from Bailet, L.L., (2001). *Development and disorders of spelling in the beginning school years*. In A.M. Bain, L.L. Bailet, & L.C. Moats, *Written language disorders: Theory into practice*, (p.30) Austin, Texas, Pro-Ed Publishers. Reprinted with permission.

**Neuropsychological Significance:** According to cognitive neuropsychology, there appear to be two distinct routes for spelling: a phonological route and one that relies on the orthographical or visual features of words (McCarthy & Warrington, 1990). In other words, some students rely on the individual sound patterns of words when spelling, while others utilize their own mental dictionary to conjure up what a given word looks like. The degree to which these two access routes are truly independent of one another has been the topic of considerable theoretical debate.

While dysphonetic spelling has been linked to lesions and/or inefficient functioning of the supramarginal gyrus, the precise anatomical location of surface dysgraphia has been a bit more elusive (Romani et. al., 1999). Nevertheless, Goldberg's (1989) gradiental model of cortical organization provides the necessary theoretical underpinnings to determine the neural wiring responsible for surface dysgraphia. To draw a comparable analogy, when Mendeleyev arranged the periodic table of elements sequentially according to their atomic weights, many elements had not yet been discovered. However, by discovering the subatomic laws by which matter was arranged, he was able to make accurate predictions about the existence of certain elements that were eventually discovered, based upon the preexisting laws of isotope measurement. Goldberg's exquisite understanding of cortical evolution provides a similar theoretical framework for mapping out cortical responsibilities, thus allowing the neuropsychologist to make reasonable assertions about cognitive functioning. According to Goldberg (1989), categorical processing is the primary function of the left hemisphere, by which language eventually evolved. From a neuroanatomical point of view, the ***angular gyrus*** lies in the gradient or intersection between the posterior portion of the parietal lobe and the occipital lobe. Therefore, along this gradient resides the seat of visual (occipital lobe) and spatial (parietal lobe) functioning of symbolic representations. Hence, surface dysgraphia can be viewed as stemming from an inability to conjure up a visual symbolic representation of a word, thereby over-relying on the phonological properties (supramargninal gyrus) of the word when spelling. It is the effective integration of these dual routes for spelling, namely the phonological and lexical routes, that leads to spelling mastery. For instance, most people need to write down a word to determine if it "looks" right in order to ensure its spelling accuracy. In truth, looking at a word on paper to determine if it matches our pre-existing image of its visual configuration is an example of the angular gyrus at work, and subsequent lexical route to spelling being deployed.

## FIGURE 4-2

### Angular gyrus and supramarginal gyrus

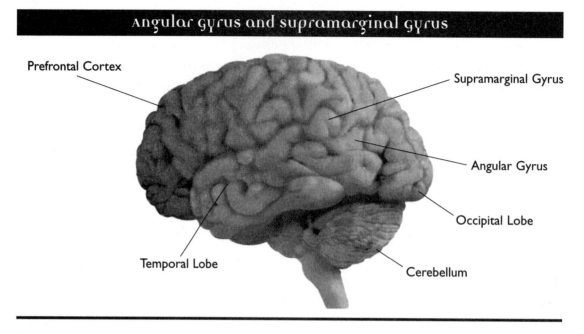

Prefrontal Cortex

Supramarginal Gyrus

Angular Gyrus

Occipital Lobe

Temporal Lobe

Cerebellum

Evidence for the neuroanatomy of the left supramarginal gyrus and left angular gyrus holding two disparate though critically important roles in the development of spelling stems from research of adults with Alzheimer's disease. There is increasing evidence to suggest a neuropsychological dissociation of writing disturbances prevalent in the early stage of Alzheimer's disease, akin to that seen in several other areas of cognition. Using PET technology, which measures glucose metabolism in the functional brain, II adults with early symptoms of Alzheimer's disease revealed highly positive correlations between metabolic ratios of the left angular gyrus with surface dysgraphia and the left supramarginal gyrus with phonological dysgraphia (Penniello, et. al., 1995). Therefore, based upon the metabolic ratios of these two distributed neural networks, two distinct routes – one phonological, the other lexical - clearly appear to underlie the writing process. Not only does this study validate the appropriateness of the neuropsychological-PET paradigms to investigate specific cognitive deficits, but it also affirms the functional utility of the cognitive gradient model to explain cortical functions.

**Mixed Dysgraphia:** Many educators often lament over students in early elementary school who make frequent reversals among letter formations in addition to reversals among letter sequences. Though letter confusion is typical among younger students in the initial stages of reading and writing, the inability to recall letter formations properly, coupled with inconsistent spelling skills, can be indicative of *mixed dysgraphia*. Often, these students demonstrate multiple perceptual deficits pertaining to word formations, rendering them vulnerable to this severe form of written language disorder. Mixed dysgraphia typically manifests itself with a combination of phonological errors when spelling, in addition to orthographic errors depicting faulty sequential arrangement of letters. There is usually little difficulty when copying written text, and generally there are well-preserved letter formation skills. However, spontaneously written sentences and words not only show misspellings, but also suffer from extra or deleted syllables or letters, making each individual word almost unrecognizable. In addition, there are often capital letters or large spaces in the middle of words, or symbols inserted that do not resemble any letter of the English alphabet (Deuel, 1995). Basically, the student has no usable key to unlocking the spelling and writing code due to multiple breakdowns subserving the written language process. Table 4-5 illustrates typical spelling miscues for students with mixed dysgraphia.

**TABLE 4-5**

| Mixed Dysgraphia Spelling Errors | | |
| --- | --- | --- |
| Target word | Misspelling | Analysis |
| advantage | advangate | letter order reversal |
| cobweb | coweb | consonant omission |
| illusion | lshn | syllable omission |
| pocket | poct | syllable omission |
| work | wrok | letter order reversal |
| kitchen | kinchen | insertion error |
| worried | werie | consonant deletion |

One of the hallmark features of mixed dysgraphia is the inability to sequence letters accurately in words. However, the number of letters in a word does not necessarily indicate the level of sophistication or degree of difficulty. For instance, the words *chaos*, *alien*, and *cohort* all contain less than seven letters but are much more challenging to spell than longer words such as *stopping*, *animals*, and *helping*, due to the phonetic irregularity of these words (Levine, 1999). Instead, effective spelling appears to depend on the ability to recall a sequence of visual and/or lexical units, depending upon the strategy one employs (Romani, et. al., 1999). The net result is one of a vast array of misspellings including additions, deletions, syllable substitutions, letter transpositions, and, in some cases, mirror or backwards writing. Unfortunately, as students pass through later grades, there is a greater demand for effective sequential synthesis of words and ideas on paper. In fact, poor sequential organization can interfere with the automatization process of reading and written language to such an extent that writing may not be available as a medium for logical thinking and reasoning (Levine, 1999).

**Neuropsychological Significance:**  In 1924, Josef Gerstmann described a patient with a series of four unusual symptoms following a left parietal stroke. The man was unable to name or identify the fingers on his hand when stimulated *(finger agnosia)*, had significant right versus left confusion, demonstrated an inability to perform mathematical operations *(acalculia)*, and exhibited significant spelling miscues when writing (Kolb & Whishaw, 1996). The errors in spelling were not attributed to a primary language disorder but rather reflected an inability to sequence letters in their appropriate order. This collection of cognitive symptoms has subsequently become entrenched in the neuropsychological literature and represents a classic clinical disorder known as **Gerstmann's Syndrome**. This disorder implicated the parietal lobes, in particular the inferior parietal lobe, as being involved in the written language process.

The functional circuitry of the left parietal lobe has been of particular interest to most educators, since this region has been associated with integrating information from visual input, and readily contributes to reading, writing, and mathematics (Kolb & Whishaw, 1996). However, the inferior parietal lobes also play an important role in the ability to learn a sequence of novel motor movements. In fact, **ideomotor apraxia**, which will be discussed in greater detail in the next chapter, refers to a disorder of motor movement in which there is an inability to copy a series of motor movements, though each individual movement can be mimicked in isolation. In other words, the disability lies in remembering sequences of stored motor engrams rather than the execution of an individual motor act. In mixed dysgraphia, part of the disorder consists of the inability to reproduce words by accurately stitching together a sequence of letters, despite having the ability to recall each letter in isolation. In a rigorous meta-analysis of PET and fMRI studies, Cabeza and Nyberg (2000) implicated the parietal lobes as having multiple functional responsibilities, with posterior parietal regions being primarily responsible for spatial perception and also involved in disengaging spatial perception. Once again, fMRI represents a recent advancement in neuroimaging, as alterations in blood flow and blood volume in activated tissue are detected, thereby permitting the study of brain functioning (Krasuski, et. al, 1996). Unlike PET scans, there is a lack of radiation and lack of invasiveness with fMRI, coupled with enhanced temporal resolution, making this the first functional technique with widespread application to children. However, given the amount of subject cooperation needed and the inability of fMRI to obtain quantitative measures of blood flow, PET still remains the gold standard for surveying the entire brain (Krasuski, et. al., 1996). In any event, a meta-analysis of more than 275 PET and fMRI studies indicated that the left parietal lobe was particularly active during verbal short-term memory tasks, holding letters in memory, and retrieving information from long-term memory (Cabeza & Nyberg, 2000). Therefore damage to the left inferior parietal lobes, which interface with the temporal and occipital lobes along the angular gyrus and supramarginal gyrus, often results in reading and written language impairments, letter distortions, and impaired spelling. Hence, mixed dysgraphia represents a more severe case of spelling and written language impairments as multiple regions along the inferior parietal regions have been implicated. However, the ability to reproduce nonverbal constructions such as drawings is often preserved (Anderson, et. al., 1993).

Perhaps no other skill requires the planning and sequential organization and arrangement of information more than written language. As will be discussed in Chapter 7, the frontal lobes play a vital role in the temporal organization of behavior and in controlling the proper sequence in which various mental operations are subsequently enacted (Goldberg, 2001). In the earliest grades, this might involve learning the days of the week, months of the year, or letters of the alphabet in a rigid order. When asked to recall what day comes after Thursday, a student might need to recite all of the days of the week until the correct answer is found. Sequential production provides an important means of organization upon which many academic tasks rely, including writing and spelling. Learning to spell through sequential analysis requires that linguistic information be preserved in a specific order to be recalled at a later date. It can be very confusing for practitioners and educators to distinguish between deficits in sequential ordering and deficits in spatial organization skills. Once again, mixed dyslexia does not necessarily involve deficits in handwriting, spacing characters on the page, copying, or visual configuration memory. Instead, tasks that involve the detection of the order of adjacent letters in a word, or the order of adjacent units in strings of consonants, or simply visual symbols appear to be at fault. (Romani et. al., 1992). Therefore, the inability to encode information in a serial order due to multiple deficits in both the inferior parietal lobule, as well as cortical connections with the prefrontal cortex, seems to be the primary neuropsychological deficit with respect to mixed dyslexia.

**Semantic/Syntactic Dysgraphia:** While most of the discussion thus far has centered on disorders of spelling, the essence of communication through print lies in the skillful assembly of words that unravel with prosaic elegance to convey a linguistic portrait of our thoughts. In fact, one could argue that the exponential growth of human intellectual prowess could be tied directly to our recent ability to permeate the boundaries of time through printed material. In other words, written language has allowed human beings to record knowledge, skills, and abilities acquired by previous generations for the use of future generations in uncovering new truths and insights. The collective knowledge base of the human species could not be accumulated without some form of documentation procedure - namely, written communication. However, an inability to master the implicit rules for grammar that dictate precisely how words and phrases can be combined lies at the heart of *semantic/syntactic dysgraphia*. There are many pitfalls to consider before a student reaches syntactic maturity, with Table 4-6 highlighting some of the main considerations:

TABLE 4-6

| written syntax disorders in print |
| --- |

- Word omissions
- Word ordering errors
- Incorrect verb and pronoun usage
- Word ending errors
- Lack of punctuation
- Lack of capitalization
- Discrepancy between oral and written language

*Adapted from Gregg, N., & Hafer, T., (2001). Disorders of Written Expression. In G.R. Lyon & J.M. Rumsey, *Neuroimaging: A window to the neurological foundations of learning and behavior in children:* (pp.111). Baltimore, MD: Paul H. Brookes Publishing Company.

The evolution of syntax in human cognitive development has been a rigorously debated topic among linguists, philosophers, anthropologists, and psychologists, all of whom examine the issue from different perspectives. It is not within the scope of this book to review these various positions and the multitude of theories that accompany each perspective. However, a brief account of the evolutionary need for the acquisition of language may shed some insight into the hierarchical structure of how language is organized and represented in our brains. Furthermore, a greater appreciation of the underlying neural architecture that contributes to the rules of symbolic thought (a notion called syntax) should assist educators in their quest to enrich the fluency of our most sophisticated linguistic endeavor to date, written language.

The prevailing notion among linguists such as Noam Chomsky remains that a language acquisition device exists solely in the human brain, thus accounting for the universality of language in all cultures, and its consistency in structure and acquisition among children. Chomsky believed words were stitched together to express a desired meaning prior to being expressed, and given the universal language similarity in all cultures, there must be a specific brain region native to humans responsible for linking spoken and written words together according to a preexisting set of rules. However, modern neuroscience has difficulty supporting this claim for a variety of reasons. First, as previously mentioned, Goldberg (1989) brilliantly deduced that the primary function of the left hemisphere was categorical processing, by which language eventually evolved, and not necessarily just a language acquisition center. In fact, the left hemisphere also processes nonlinguistic representations such as sequences, colors, and various emotional states (Damasio, 1999). Second, there is no evidence for an individual language center in the brain, as one of the more compelling features of neuralinguistic representations remains the vast distribution of language centers throughout the cortex. Third, by most accounts, the appreciation of music takes place in the right hemisphere with most trained musicians having as much as 25 percent more cortical tissue in the right temporal lobe as opposed to the left temporal lobe (Carter, 1998). Many initial communicative forms, customs, and rituals stemmed from musical sounds, whether to signal warnings of impending danger or to serve as a beacon to a specific deity. Certainly, music served as an early communicative device through chants, beats, and harmony, with the neural underpinnings of this particular sound based classification system taking place independent of language and in the opposite hemisphere.

Still, there is much validity to the general premise of Chomsky's argument for a genetic underpinning of language acquisition, for no other reason than children cannot possibly be taught each and every rule necessary for language production and comprehension. Consider this: by the time we graduate from high school, the 44 phonemes that constitute the English language can be combined and arranged to form some 45,000 to 60,000 recognizable words. This massive lexicon of words can be further combined into sentences and paragraphs, and eventually used as a medium for reasoning, problem solving, and persuasion. Thus, the human brain must be preset in some capacity that allows us to extract rules for word combinations based upon the prevailing speech patterns from our environment. The question of how remains a topic for continued scholarly debate, but it invites a closer look.

Fossils reveal that the earliest *Homo sapiens* appeared some 100,000 to 200,000 years ago, with the general consensus being that the fast-paced symbolic language that we use in our speech today has existed for the past 50,000 years (Ratey, 2001). Perhaps the evolutionary need for cognitive compression was spawned somewhere in our lineage. In other words, language was an evolutionary necessity to categorize our expanding knowledge structure of the world. Through an economy of thought, one symbol such as the word "*rock*" could now encapsulate many theoretical representations such as its visual description, its firmness, or its use as a tool or weapon under a single semantic category.

According to Damasio (1999), language seemed to evolve ***after*** human beings had become adept at categorizing actions and creating mental representations of objects, events, and relations. Even linguistic scholars such as Derek Bickerton and James Hurford (2000) agree that syntactic structures evolve at least in part on the basis of pre-existing semantic representations. The computational models of Hurford are consistent with Bickerton's view, as they assume mental representational structures predated communication, which then gave rise to linguistic structures. Thus, embedded within our neural circuitry and perhaps forever interwoven within the structural nature of our cortex lies a neural progression first of motoric categories, then gestures, sequences of gestures to communicate, and finally linguistic concepts. Consequently, the left hemisphere initially began to communicate through simple motor sequences and gestures, then the brain eventually evolved to the point that a sound-based classification system accompanying these gestures was laid down. In fact, the link between speech and movement can be seen in babies (Ratey, 2001). Long before they start talking, babies become skilled at using eye contact, facial expressions, and nonverbal gestures to communicate. Most skilled parents even become accustomed to certain pitches of cooing and crying that correspond to eating, drinking, sleeping, and bathroom patterns. The following chapter will expound upon the relationship between sequencing and planning motor skills and oral and written language development. However, Table 4-7 reveals the basic components universally observed in sound-based language systems.

# TABLE 4-7

## components of a sound based language system

**Phonemes** - the individual sound units that produce morphemes. The English language consists of 44 phonemes.

**Morphemes** - the smallest meaningful units of a word, whose subsequent combination creates individual words.

**Syntax** - the rules of grammar that allow for the meaningful combinations of words in phrases and sentences.

**Lexicon** - the collection of all words in a given language. Each lexical entity includes all information with morphological or syntactical rules.

**Semantics** - the meanings that correspond to all lexical items and words.

**Prosody** - the vocal intonations that can modify the literal meaning of words and sentences.

**Discourse** - the linking of sentences in order to constitute a narrative.

Since all writing systems are comprised of symbols, syntax dictates the structure by which the infinite number of combinations of semantic concepts can be arranged to organize our thoughts effectively and communicate them with others. Although chimpanzees can learn to name objects in a manner at a similar rate to babies, they cannot develop a set of rules that allow them to combine signs and express their ideas or intuitions (Ratey, 2001). To summarize, language reflects the ability to represent objects in the external world through symbols. Linguistic concepts stem from mental representations that were first expressed through motoric gestures, eye contact, and nonverbal communication methodologies prior to a sound-based system of classification being established.

The brain has always been an organ of cognitive economy, and to appreciate more complex concepts fully, a system of grammatical rules was established to link, combine, and reformulate semantic principles in an infinite capacity. Therefore, the brain appears to have three distinct mechanisms for processing language, each of which is relatively independent of one another and constitutes different brain regions. *Phonological* processing evaluates the sequence of sounds, with deficits generally resulting in reading and spelling difficulties. *Syntactic* processing involves the embedded rules that dictate how words are combined, with deficits resulting in semantic/syntactic dysgraphia. Lastly, *semantic* processing refers to the meaningful concept displayed by the combination of words expressed according to the rules of syntax. For instance, the sentence "bitten the dog hurt his finger boy" violates both syntactic and semantic rules, assuming that the original intent was to say, "The boy hurt his finger when he was bitten by the dog."

Since errors in syntax also lead to imprecise errors in meaning, the term semantic/syntactic dysgraphia has been coined to reflect these specific deficits.

In our schools today, we see children who display extreme difficulty conveying meaning through print due to a breakdown in their knowledge of linguistic rules. Teachers sometimes appear at a loss to assist children in their attempts to write because it remains a bit unclear as to the precise nature of how syntax evolved in the first place. In other words, the question is whether writing can actually be taught so that basic principles of syntactical development can be generalized to the tens of thousands of words in the lexicon of a child. In fact, little research can be found in the literature to support the explicit teaching of grammar rules as a means of improving compositional skills, as it appears the teaching of grammar in isolation does not serve any practical purpose (Hillocks & Smith, 1991). However, cognitive neuroscience is breaking the shackles of linking a unitary deficit with a unitary brain function, thus redefining educational methodologies to fit with the concept of multiple brain systems that constitute a specific function. In other words, by understanding the hierarchical organization and development of language within the brain, most linguistic errors are indeed correctable, even in skills as complex and sophisticated as written language (Ratey, 2001).

**Neuropsychological Significance:** Approximately 150 years ago, Pierre Paul Broca and Carl Wernicke discovered the rough location of basic language centers in the brain. Wernicke determined that cortical regions in the left *superior temporal gyrus* seem to be responsible for the understanding of language for 99 percent of right-handers and 70 percent of left-handers. This led to the concept of *cerebral dominance*, which referred to language being lateralized in the left hemisphere of most individuals. Interestingly, handedness also seemed to be intertwined with language dominance, lending further credence to the theory that motoric gestures being sequentially called upon to communicate basic concepts were a general precursor to vocal language development. In any event, damage to this region resulted in *Wernicke's Aphasia*, or the inability to comprehend speech. Conversely, damage to Broca's area in the prefrontal cortex resulted in *Broca's Aphasia*, or the inability to produce speech when comprehension is preserved. However, the language system as represented in the brain is somewhat more complicated than this simple dichotomy.

The seeds of the neural representation of language in present-day humans were sown in our distant evolutionary past. According to Goldberg (1989), most language representations are multimodal, though certain classes of words such as nouns are more likely to be represented in the cortical areas involved with visual processing. After all, nouns represent concrete objects such as *table, chair, strawberry*, or *shirt* that can be readily observed and visualized. On the other hand, the cerebral representation of verbs is housed closer to the motor regions in the anterior portion of the brain, or premotor cortex. Once again, verbs such as *play, run, deliver,* or *send* all denote some sort of action to be taken. As mentioned before, the brain has a knack for a certain level of cognitive efficiency when processing information, and through evolution, the mental representations of the physical world became more economically stored when housed geographically by its corresponding sensory modality. Therefore, the cerebral representation of semantic knowledge is not compact, but rather distributed throughout the cortex (Damasio, 1999)

## FIGURE 4-3

**noun and verb distribution in the brain**

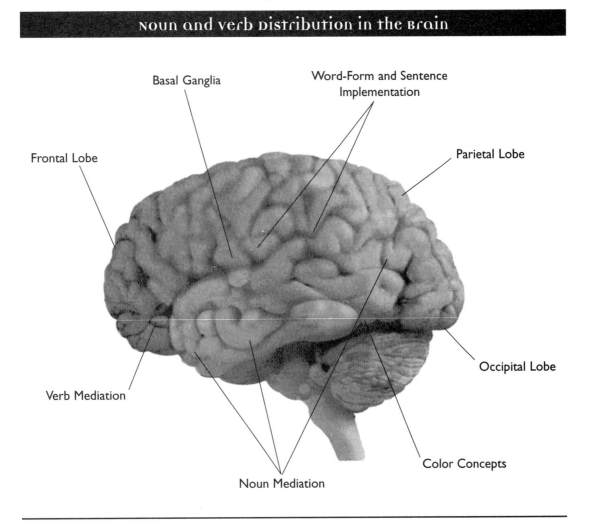

*Adapted from Damasio, A.R., (1999). The scientific American book of the brain. New York: The Lyons Press.*

The notion that specific categories of language are distributed throughout the brain represents a marked paradigm shift away from Chomsky's original search for a language activation device in the cortex. Furthermore, some of the more remarkable findings among students with dysgraphia can now be conceptualized and more readily explained. For instance, *deep dysgraphia* is a subtype of semantic/syntactic dysgraphia whereby students have little difficulty spelling nouns or highly familiar words but make significant semantic substitution errors when writing. In other words, the content of their writing passages often lacks cohesion and unity of thought, with only highly familiar nouns spelled correctly.

Jenni Ogden (1996) noticed that adults who had their entire left hemisphere removed to relieve intractable seizures, a procedure known as a hemipherectomy, showed signs of deep dysgraphia. She reasoned that the remaining right hemisphere was somewhat feeble in its attempt to read and write and was not capable of phonological processing. Thus, whole word recognition of words, usually by sight, was the only means attainable to determine meaning from print. Familiar nouns that tended to conjure up a visual image were more easily identified since they tend to be housed near the occipital lobes, or vision centers, of the brain. Thus, orthographic or visual cues could be utilized to retrieve this category of words. However, more abstract words that do not necessarily conjure up a visual image, such as *ideology* or *reconnaissance*, could not be identified since they were located in other regions throughout the cortex. Consequently, the right hemisphere had no way to retrieve these words since it was incapable of using phonological cues as a retrieval strategy. Studies by Baxter & Warrington (1985) also noted this type of category-specific dysgraphia. Their research confirmed that nouns were recalled and spelled more accurately than adjectives, and adjectives were recalled and spelled more accurately than verbs. Thus, concrete words that humans can easily image in their minds can be retrieved by more visual means, though more abstract words and verbs tend to be organized in a manner whereby phonological or sound-symbol cues are needed for retrieval.

Frequent semantic substitution errors when writing are a second component of deep dysgraphia. Once again, much imprecision seems to exist when attempting to write words from specific semantic categories when the left hemisphere is not involved (Ogden, 1995). For instance, when attempting to write the sentence, "*He used a spoon when eating,*" the wrong word in a given semantic category may become activated, yielding a sentence such as, "*He used a fork when drinking.*" Deep dysgraphia is often a double-deficit type of dysgraphia characterized by marked impairments in spelling non-words and phonologically irregular words, in addition to frequent semantic errors and substitutions when writing.

Research by Moro et. al. (2001) has indicated that the left hemisphere is chiefly involved with syntactical processing. In particular, the region around Broca's area allows for sentence word order to be checked, stored, and retrieved, and is very much involved in the hierarchical syntactic structure of language. However, the syntactic capacities of the brain are not entirely located in a single area, but rather involve both hemispheres as well as other portions of the brain, including the basal ganglia and the cerebellum. The functional importance of the basal ganglia and the cerebellum will be highlighted in Chapter 5, though both regions are involved with the automaticity and fluency of motor responses, and participate in complex planning (Goldberg, 2001). Therefore, the areas of the brain responsible for stitching together the tens of thousands of words stored throughout the cortex in a coherent syntactical fashion appear to lie within various regions of the frontal lobes centered around Broca's area. Figure 4-4 illustrates the various brain regions being activated during different linguistic tasks, further evidencing the vast distribution of neural networks involved in language.

## FIGURE 4-4

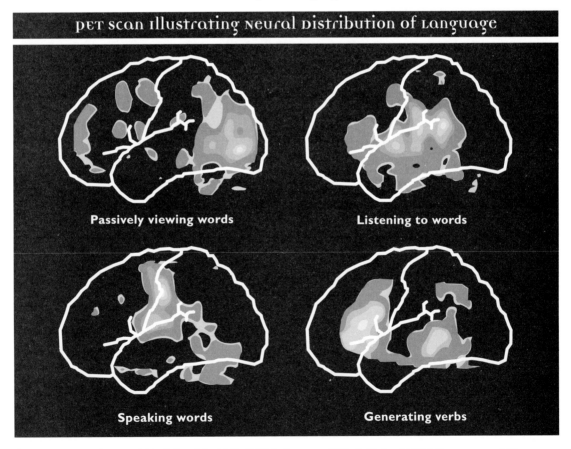

**PET SCAN ILLUSTRATING NEURAL DISTRIBUTION OF LANGUAGE**

Passively viewing words

Listening to words

Speaking words

Generating verbs

*Adapted from Posner, M.I., & Raichle, M.E., (1994). *Images of Mind.* Oxford: W.H. Freeman and Company.

# subtypes of Non-Language Based Dysgraphias

## Chapter 5

"without a struggle, there can be no progress"
— frederick Douglass

Though the literature is rife with research analysis on how human thought becomes symbolically represented though print, there has been far less emphasis on the physical act of constructing print, the process known as handwriting. Most educators and parents at the early elementary grades often denounce the tenacious nature of handwriting difficulties in children, and cite poor motivation and carelessness as the underlying cause of messy work. Since computers have become more prevalent as educational tools and devices for interactive learning, the simple punch of a keystroke or click of a mouse can circumvent fine motor sloppiness in print. Still, motor actions such as typing on a keyboard, swinging a golf club, or manipulating a pencil involve a specific sequence of muscular actions, or what Luria described as motor engrams, which are stored patterns of familiar *motor actions*. Luria (1980) described handwriting as ideas with purpose and action that are translated into specific visual and kinesthetic programs stored in the form of motor engrams. As mentioned previously, a survey of fine-motor activity requirements in elementary schools in Massachusetts showed that 30% to 60% of the time in school was spent mostly in fine-motor activity (Deuel, 1995).

Furthermore, considerably more time is spent during the preschool years as students focus on coloring, tracing, using scissors, and drawing in order to develop appropriate readiness skills for future writing skills to commence.

The degree to which graphomotor output problems directly impact written language skills remains a topic of considerable debate (Burton & Dancisak, 2000). Nevertheless, the emergent field of school occupational therapy has exploded onto the special educational scene, with millions of dollars spent toward reconciling fine motor output difficulty in children. By all accounts, occupational therapy remains a valuable resource for children either to remediate fine motor deficits or to retrain students through augmentative technology to function more independently in the classroom. The Schneck and Henderson (1990) scale, depicted in Table 5-1, remains the gold standard in the evaluation of developmental grip progressions in children. The first five grips, as depicted in Figure 5-1, were labeled *primitive*, since they were rarely seen in children after age four. The next three grips were deemed *transitional* since they decrease with age, though they still may persist beyond age six. The final two grips represent *mature grips*, as there is a permanence maintained into adulthood. Schneck (1991) further combined similar grips within a 5-point level system, and noted that children with writing difficulties obtained significantly lower mean grip scores (4.70) than other children (4.93).

## fIGURE 5-1

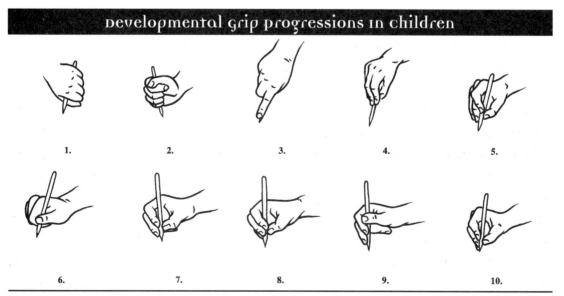

### Developmental grip progressions in children

1.   2.   3.   4.   5.

6.   7.   8.   9.   10.

*Adapted from Schneck, C.M., & Henderson, A., (1990). Descriptive analysis of the developmental progression of grip position for pencil and crayon control in nondysfunctional children. *American Journal of Occupational Therapy*, 44, 893-900.

## TABLE 5-1

| Grip Number[a] | Grip Level Number[b] | Description |
|---|---|---|
| 1 | 1 | Radial cross palmar grasp; implement positioned across palm radially {thumb down}; implement held with fisted hand; forearm fully pronated; full arm movement |
| 2 | 2 | Palmar supinate grasp; implement positioned across palm projecting ulnarly {thumb up}; implement held with fisted hand; wrist slightly flexed and supinated away from midposition; full arm movement |
| 3 | 2 | Digital pronate grasp, only index finger extended: implement held in palmar grasp; index finger extended along pencil toward tip, arm not supported on table; full arm movement |
| 4 | 3 | Brush grasp: implement held with fingers; earser end positioned against palm; hand pronated with wrist movement present; whole arm movement; forearm positioned in air |
| 5 | 3 | Grasp with extended fingers: implement held with fingers; wrist straight and pronated with slight ulnar deviation; forearm moves as a unit |
| 6 | 4 | Cross thumb grasp: fingers fisted loosely into palm; implement held against index finger; thumb crossed over pencil toward index finger; finger and wrist movement; forearm positioned on table |
| 7 | 4 | Static tripod grasp: implement stabilized against radial side of third digit by thumb pulp; index pulp on top of shaft; thumb stabilized in full opposition; wrist slightly extended; hand moves as a unit; implement rests in open web space; forearm resting on table |
| 8 | 4 | Four fingers grasp: implement held with four fingers in opposition; wrist and finger movement; forearm positioned on table |

| 9 | 5 | Lateral tripod grasp: implement stabilized against radial side of third digit by thumb pulp; index pulp on top of shaft of implement; thumb adducted and braced over or under anywhere along lateral border of index finger; wrist slightly extended; fourth and fifth digits flexed to stabilize the metacarpophalangeal arch and third digit; localized movements of digits of tripod and wrist movements on tall and horizontal strokes; forearm resting on table |
|---|---|---|
| 10 | 5 | Dynamic tripod grasp: implement stabilized against radial side of third digit by thumb pulp; index pulp on top of shaft of implement; thumb stabilized in full opposition; wrist slightly extended; fourth and fifth digits flexed to stabilize the metacarpophalangeal arch and third digit; localized movements of digits of tripod and wrist movements on tall and horizontal strokes; forearm resting on table |

[a]Adapted from Schneck, C.M., & Henderson, A., (1990). Descriptive analysis of the developmental progression of grip position for pencil and crayon control in nondysfunctional children. American Journal of Occupational Therapy, 44, 893-900. [b]Adapted from Schneck, C.M., (1991). Comparison of pencil-grip patterns in first graders with food and poor handwriting skills. American Journal of Occupational Therapy, 45, 701-706.

The tripod posture has traditionally been viewed as the most effective pencil grip, though idiosyncratic representations of this grip do not necessarily result in less effective or inaccurate graphomotor performance (Burton & Dancisak, 2000). Still, children who perform at the lower end of the accuracy scale are the ones most likely to be treated by occupational therapists, and may be able to improve their writing and drawing accuracy by modifying their grip. In addition, forearm position plays a vital role in the extent of the writing process, perhaps more so than a specific grip or pressure. Lastly, any grip, whether efficient or inefficient, tends to become kinesthetically *locked in* so that changing a child's grasp pattern at certain ages may not be a viable option.

**Ideomotor Apraxia**  The generic term *apraxia* refers to a wide variety of motor skill deficits in which the voluntary execution of a skilled motor movement is impaired. By definition, this impairment is not the result of paralysis, paresis, or lack of comprehension. The defining feature of *ideomotor apraxa* is the failure to carry out a motor act or gesture on verbal command, even though comprehension is preserved and the motor skills necessary to perform the command are intact (Filley, 1995). Nevertheless, the same motor skill act can be effectively executed if done so in a spontaneous manner. For instance, when asked to wave good-bye or imitate drinking a glass of water, a student may fail to generate any response, persevere with another motor response, or simply use vocalizations as opposed to the desired motor action (Filley, 1995). However, in the course of play or in some other type of spontaneous situation these gestures may be performed with little difficulty. Ideomotor apraxia refers to a single action, not a sequence of actions such as those necessary to manipulate a pencil when writing a lengthy passage.

There are multiple brain regions and neural networks responsible for organizing, planning, and executing motor skill functions. Just as language appears to be represented in various regions of the brain in a certain hierarchical fashion, motor skill functioning is housed in a similar fashion. According to Ratey (2001), the neural distribution of motor skill functioning is analogous to a two-story house. The basement level represents the original structure or foundation that is critical to the formation and design of the rest of the house. The basement level of our motor system is the autonomic nervous system consisting of the brain stem and spinal cord. This level is not under conscious awareness and is responsible for maintaining basic bodily functions such as heartbeat, respiration, and other internal organs. Signals are constantly relayed to the hypothalamus as the two reciprocal branches of this system, the sympathetic and parasympathetic nervous system, work in tandem to keep the body in the right balance. The first floor of our motor system consists of the *basal ganglia* and *cerebellum*, both of which involve binding together a series of complex motor movements into a smooth and coordinated activity. The *cerebellum* has been implicated specifically in the timing of muscle movements, in addition to being involved with body balance and accuracy of specific movements (Kolb & Whishaw, 1996). The *basal ganglia*, located subcortically in the forebrain, have no direct connections with the spinal cord, though they weigh heavily in the automaticity of motor skill functioning in the absence of cognitive awareness. For instance, when riding a bicycle, driving a car, or performing any *over-learned* task, the basal ganglia play a crucial role in procuring these tasks in order to free up cognitive workspace and energy for other endeavors. Often, commuters become so cognitively entrenched in the forthcoming activities of their day that driving to work is almost an automatic response. Frequent comments such as "*I arrived to work on time, but have no recollection of my drive.*" are not atypical. Much appreciation should be given toward the role of the basal ganglia for serving as a motor skills autopilot.

Perhaps signing one's name remains the only aspect of written language activity that actually becomes over-learned and therefore capable of being under the command of the basal ganglia. For most adults and especially professional athletes who routinely sign on a daily basis, the sheer repetitiveness of this mundane act often becomes subserved by more subcortical functions, as little conscious awareness is needed. Though each signature is unique, there remains surprising consistency among them, so much that banks and other institutions frequently check the authenticity of this written act as a means of proper identification. Using functional magnetic resonance imaging (fMRI), researchers (Scholz, et. al., 2000) noted that the left basal ganglia was primarily responsible for controlling over-learned motor engrams such as writing one's name, in part by inhibiting other competing motor movements. Furthermore, the right basal ganglia appeared more active when learning a new motor task, such as finger tapping or toe tapping, though once the task was mastered, the left basal ganglia took command of the process (Scholz, et. al., 2000). This type of hemispheric specialization is consistent with Goldberg's (1989) theory that the right hemisphere, with its increased density in white matter, appeared more suited toward novel stimuli, while the left hemisphere, with its increased density in gray matter, appeared tailored toward more routinized information.

The second or top floor of our motor skills' house consists of the motor strip and pre-motor cortex that comprise the posterior portion of the frontal lobes. The *primary motor cortex* or motor strip is the physical representation of our limbs and body parts in our brain, with the mouth, hands, and genitalia being over-represented. The *pre-motor cortex* is very much analogous to the band conductor instructing the band (motor cortex) what to do and when to do it. In other words, the pre-motor cortex instructs the motor cortex when to execute a specific task. Ideomotor apraxia may also be seen in deep parietal-frontal connections and/or input to callosal pathways. Feedback is vitally important, much as the conductor listens for subtle nuances of how the orchestra (the body) is doing and makes continuous adjustments to speed up or slow down (Ratey, 2001). Therefore, in the case of ideomotor apraxia, there is often damage to the left pre-motor cortex inhibiting the conductor's ability to direct the orchestra, or damage to the *arcuate fasciculus*, which prevents the instructor from monitoring the feedback (proprioception) of the orchestra (Filley, 1995). The band itself remains intact, but the synchrony and harmony of each musician is off-key. If a certain skill such as waving good-bye has become automatized, then the first floor or basal ganglia can take the reins. In summary, the pre-motor cortex is vital for the conscious ability to direct motor movement, though spontaneous movement not under complete conscious awareness can be subserved by lower brain regions - but not necessarily on command.

## FIGURE 5-2

**Frontal Lobe Subdivisions**

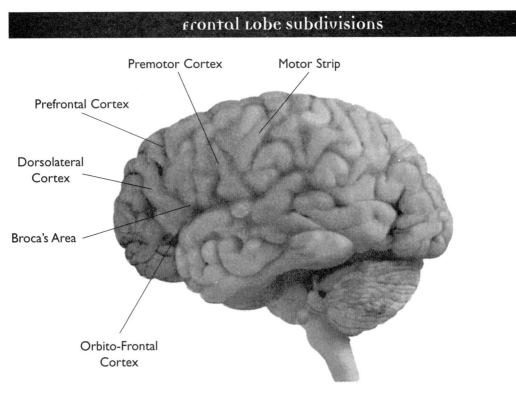

Premotor Cortex

Motor Strip

Prefrontal Cortex

Dorsolateral Cortex

Broca's Area

Orbito-Frontal Cortex

Since some aspects of language such as phonology are represented differently in males and females (See Chapter 4), and since there is a strong correlation between motor skill selection and speech, then it stands to reason that perhaps some degree of differentiation in motor skill dysfunction exists between male and female brains. Kimura (1999) stumbled upon such differences in working with patients with left hemispheric damage due to stroke. It appeared as though damage to more anterior brain regions resulted in ideomotor apraxia for women, though damage to more posterior regions resulted in the same apraxia for men. In essence, women's motor selection system was located in closer proximity to the motor cortex, thus allowing for greater enhancement of fine motor skills. Perhaps this is why most teachers generally believe that little girls have more precise handwriting skills than boys. In contrast, men's motor skill selection system seemed housed in more posterior left hemispheric regions, closer to the occipital cortex that processes vision. This region is closer in proximity to more spatially oriented regions, which may explain why boys tend to be more skilled in visual-spatial endeavors. Figure 5-3 depicts regions in the male and female brain most susceptible to apraxia. It should be noted that Goldberg (2001) has argued quite persuasively that differences between male and female brains are more related to anterior/posterior organizational attributes, as opposed to left vs. right hemispheric attributes.

## fIGURE 5-3

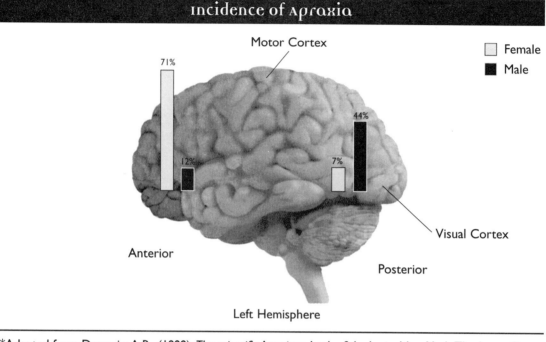

**Incidence of Apraxia**

Motor Cortex

71%

12%

44%

7%

☐ Female
■ Male

Anterior

Visual Cortex

Posterior

Left Hemisphere

*Adapted from Damasio, A.R., (1999). *The scientific American book of the brain.* New York: The Lyons Press.

**Ideational Apraxia:** Virtually every aspect of writing has a sequential component. The formation of individual letters requires sequential activation of a series of motor engrams, while the careful selection of words to convey a thought process properly remains a writer's greatest challenge. The term ideational apraxia refers to a failure in performing a sequential motor act, though each individual act can be performed in isolation and on command. For instance, a series of actions such as folding a letter, inserting the letter in an envelope, sealing the envelope, and then placing a stamp on it remains difficult, despite the fact that each individual act can be executed (Filley, 1995). Therefore, performing a sequentially driven task such as written language remains highly problematic for students with ideational apraxia, despite the preservation of individual letter formation skills. For these children, writing is often slow and laborious, and characterized by frequently erasing, correcting, or crossing out one's writing. The ability to copy is often preserved, though prone to careless errors (O'Hare & Brown, 1989). Once again, the most salient feature of this type of apraxia is the inability to sequence a chain of motor acts. Figure 5-4 illustrates an example of a student attempting to copy a sentence with ideational apraxia.

FIGURE 5-4

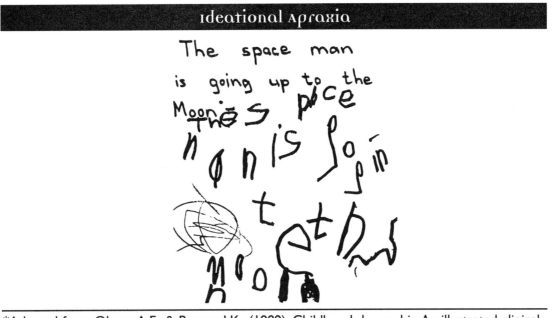

ideational Apraxia

*Adapted from Ohare, A.E., & Brown, J.K., (1989). Childhood dysgraphia: An illustrated clinical classification. *Child Care Health Development,* 15(2), 79-104. Printed with permission.

Quite often, teachers lament about the sheer difficulty students experience when initiating a written language activity. Both teachers and parents are often frustrated over the amount of time taken to complete a written classroom or homework assignment in an independent manner. However, any sequential production of information generally requires some form of prior sequential organization. Since students with ideational apraxia often lack the necessary organization skills to foresee a stepwise progression of events from beginning to middle to end, they tend to become stuck or entrenched in their efforts to produce written language. In addition, these students frequently have time management problems in the classroom, as there is no capacity to allocate time in appropriate increments to complete activities requiring multiple steps (Levine, 1999). Learning through sequential analysis, from memorizing the steps in long division, to synchronizing motor movements in swinging a golf club, to the development of written language syntax, requires that we preserve some type of serial order.

According to Van Galen (1991) there are three specific processing components required to complete a given motor task. With respect to writing, the following psychomotor steps are deployed: (1) **Motor Programming,** or the retrieval of learned motor engrams from long-term memory; (2) **Muscular Initiation,** the process of recruiting motor neurons necessary to perform a desired motor activity, which plays an important role in the consistency of a motor act; and (3) *Parameterization,* which is the proprioceptive feedback mechanism that allows for the regulation of the overall force, tempo, and rhymicity of a task. This might include modulating letter formation quality, size, slant control, and pencil holding postures. Since ideational apraxia primarily occurs with damage to the left hemisphere (Kolb & Whishaw, 1996), there must be a specific brain region responsible for integrating and modulating the motor skills necessary for written output. Research by Anderson et. al. (1993) has implicated **Exner's** area in the left dorsolateral frontal lobe as being responsible for the convergence of many aspects of the writing process. This area appears to have a unique capacity for coordinated sequential activation of stored representations, and is richly interconnected with primary motor cortices to recruit motor neurons in the dominant arm and hand. Furthermore, there are strong interconnections with language-related cortices, thus allowing for the sequential activation of visual-motor units linked with linguistic knowledge.

## fIGURE 5-5

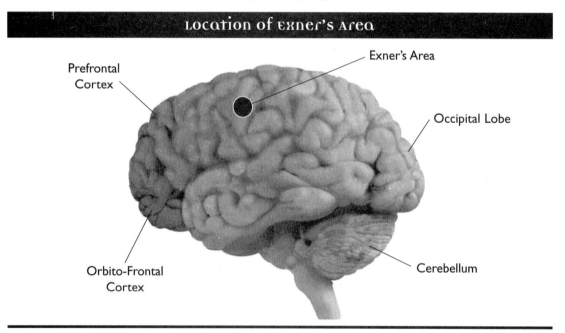

### Location of Exner's Area

Since written language is a multifaceted phenomenon, the notion of a specific brain region responsible for integrating all the neural components of the writing process is intuitively appealing, though perhaps a bit simplistic. As noted previously, through evolution there has been a certain division of labor within the brain with the left hemisphere more inclined toward processing routine-oriented, over-learned information and the right hemisphere more disposed toward processing novel stimuli

(Goldberg & Costa, 1981). Hence, there must be some sort of transfer from the right hemisphere to the left for the eventual mastery and automaticity of a given task. Since ideational apraxia involves a fundamental breakdown of the sequential arrangement of a series of *previously* learned and acquired motor tasks, the left hemisphere obviously becomes implicated. In summary, the left hemisphere plays a vital role in processing information with pre-existing structures such as verbal information for speech or motor engrams for writing. Consequently, there is tremendous overlap between a specific lesion to the left hemisphere producing either aphasia (disorders of speech) and/or apraxia (disorder of motor movement). Thus, sequential fine motor skill development and linguistic abilities, both of which rely on the ability to link multiple motor or linguistic skills, stem from similar neural mechanisms forever intertwined though evolution.

**Constructional Dyspraxia:** While much of the discussion has focused on the role of the left hemisphere with respect to written language abilities, one must also consider the exact contribution of the right hemisphere. Since only human beings have brains with two hemispheres that differ so radically in structure and function, it would appear as though higher-level, sophisticated learning necessitates some level of functional independence between the hemispheres. After all, the right hemisphere must deal with most initial or novel stages of learning on some level, prior to information being transferred to the left hemisphere. According to Ramachandran (1998), each hemisphere not only possesses different roles and specializations, but also interprets the world in a manner diametrically opposed to the other. For instance, the left hemisphere actually *creates* its own belief system and attempts to fold new information into its pre-existing model of the world. Similar to conservative sects of most religions, the left hemisphere will deny, repress, or fabricate bits of reality in a desperate attempt to preserve its world view and pre-existing biases. On the other hand, the right hemisphere offers the perfect counterbalance by questioning the status quo and actually attempting to find cognitive inconsistencies. Analogous to an agnostic sect of most religions, its job is to question aspects of reality to such an extent that our comprehension and subsequent world view must change to accommodate new exceptions to the rule.

With respect to written language, the right hemisphere certainly has some very important linguistic capabilities, most of which are centered on gauging the emotional color of cognitive events. For instance, determining the emotional state of words from the tone of the speaker or comprehending metaphor and humor appear to fall under the purview of the non-dominant or right hemisphere. Though the right hemisphere can comprehend spoken or written concepts, it certainly possesses significant limitations, as it cannot speak or spell (Ogden, 1996). According to Ratey (2001), there are significant limitations of the left hemisphere with regard to language functions, which become surprisingly obvious upon damage to the right hemisphere. For instance, following a right hemispheric stroke, language is often interpreted in a literal fashion and there is much difficulty comprehending the emotional tones of speech and regulating prosody. In fact, many of the problematic language skills often seen with high functioning autistic students are rather similar to this condition, as there is no counterbalance to the left hemisphere's predisposition to view the world in a linear and concrete manner. In terms of written language prowess, deficits in right hemisphere functioning tend to produce rather mechanistic writing, void of the rich emotional tones that color language. In addition, there is usually much brevity and a lack of output in creative writing, as a sparingly limited amount of words are used to convey factual events in a rote fashion. Certainly, this can be an asset for technical writers and secretaries summing up dictation in shorthand, but it often poses significant limitations for the more prosaic compositions often required in academic settings. Still, the hallmark feature of faulty right hemispheric functioning with respect to written language is the fundamental breakdown of the visual spatial synthesis of written production; a disorder referred to as **constructional dyspraxia**. Table 5-3 lists the differences between left and right parietal lobe functioning with respect to learning.

## TABLE 5-3

### Differential Functioning of Left vs. Right Parietal Lobes

I. **Left Parietal Lesions:**
  (a) Dyslexia – reading impairment
  (b) Dysgraphia – written language impairment
  (c) Astereognosis – inability to name objects by touch using right hand.
  (d) Ideomotor apraxia – inability to sequence motor skills
  (e) Gerstmann's Syndrome – right/left confusion, math & written language difficulty.
  (f) Various aphasic disorders – speech impairments

II. **Right Parietal Lesions:**
  (a) Constructional dyspraxia – visual-motor deficits
  (b) Geographic disorientation – spatial deficits
  (c) Astereognosis – inability to name objects by touch using left hand.
  (d) Dyscalculia – math deficits due to inability to line up numbers appropriately.
  (e) Denial or neglect of left side of page.

* Adapted from Strub, R.L., & Black, F.W., (1992). Neurobehavioral disorders: A clinical approach (p.282).

According to Smits-Engelsman & Van Galen (1997), poor handwriting skills stem not from a failure of the motor programming process of production, but rather from an overwhelming failure to obey spatial constraints coupled with a lack of consistency. In essence, the failure to control spatial accuracy was the most salient discriminating feature between students with good and poor handwriting skills. Contrary to popular belief, there really was little evidence that poor handwriting was a transient developmental delay, and that children may eventually outgrow their sloppy written language patterns over time. Therefore, constructional dyspraxia represents an inability to produce and/or modulate written language production due to deficits with the spatial constraints of letter and word production. Figures 5-6 and 5-7 illustrate the inherent difficulty for both teachers and parents in interpreting this type of written language impairment.

## FIGURE 5-6

### constructional dyspraxia

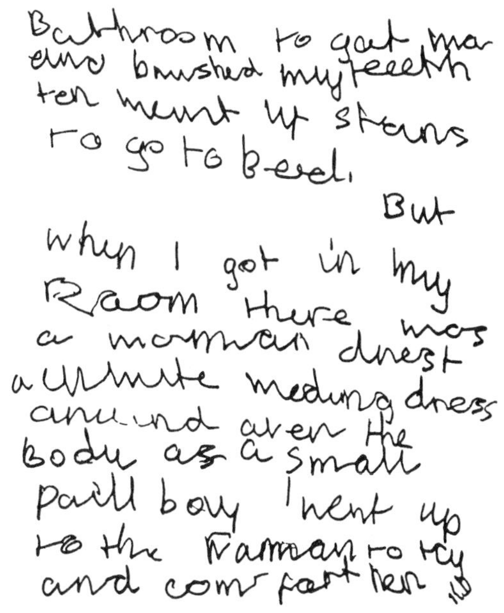

*Adapted from Ohare, A.E., & Brown, J.K., (1989). Childhood dysgraphia: An illustrated clinical classification. *Child Care Health Development,* 15(2), 79-104. Printed with permission.

## FIGURE 5-7

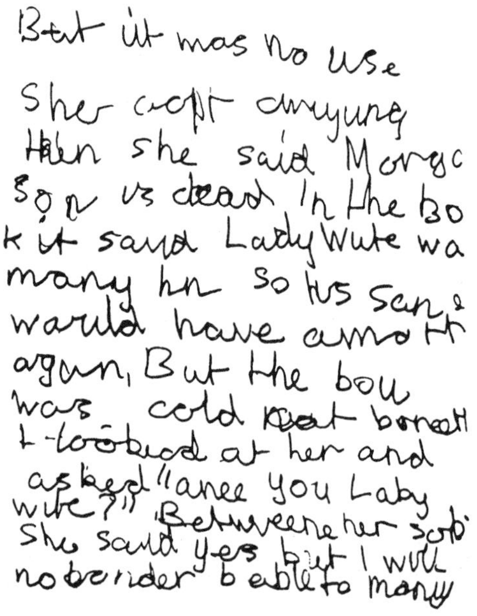

*Adapted from Ohare, A.E., & Brown, J.K., (1989). Childhood dysgraphia: An illustrated clinical classification. *Child Care Health Development,* 15(2), 79-104. Printed with permission.

The assessment of visual-motor integration skills, or constructional dyspraxia, has become a permanent fixture in most psychological evaluations. However, popular measures such as the *Bender-Gestalt* initially emerged to assist in the diagnosis of dyslexia. For the better part of the 20th century, the work of Samuel Orton (1925) and Maryann Frostig (1968) popularized the notion that students who reversed letters, such as *"b"* for *"d"*, were harboring faulty visual perceptual skills and inadequate cerebral dominance for linguistic skills. In other words, Orton, revered by most educators as the father of learning disabilities, determined that reversals were the by-product of competing messages sent by the normally docile right hemisphere that prevented the left hemisphere from accurately detecting linguistic information from print. Fueled by Frostig's notion that reading was primarily a visual perceptual task, numerous visual-motor training exercises were developed to treat problematic reading and written language skills in children and re-establish the left hemisphere's dominant role. Despite neuropsychology's efforts to underscore that reading and written language were primarily linguistic tasks, with deficits generally implicating multiple brain regions along the perisylvian region, remnants of this old paradigm remain entrenched in popular psychology. As will be discussed in the following chapter, letter reversals are primarily the by-product of a faulty grapheme buffer, and not the residual effects of the right hemisphere being far too engaged in the reading and writing process. However, virtually every test battery administered by psychologists still includes a test of visual-motor integration.

Still, the importance of copying cannot be underscored enough with respect to integrating the visual-motor pathways necessary for written language production. Most young children learn to write by copying shapes, drawing pictures, emulating numbers and letters, and eventually learning to write their first names. As noted previously, the left hemisphere eventually subserves the writing process, but in the initial stages of learning, the visual-motor representations of objects in space are primarily a right hemisphere event. In fact, many studies of functional magnetic resonance imaging (fMRI) have illustrated that copying letters in virtually any language is mediated by the right superior parietal lobe (Matsuo, et. al., 2000). On the other hand, writing to dictation, a process utilizing the auditory input of information, seems to be mediated by Broca's area in the left frontal cortex, a region vital to the production of speech (Matsuo, et. al., 2000). Perhaps in some cases, the overzealous left hemisphere takes command of the writing process prior to the right hemisphere effectively synthesizing visual-spatial representations of print, thus leading to sloppy, though automatically consistent, handwriting. This may explain why artists, many of whom have well developed visual-spatial cortices in the right hemisphere (Carter, 1998), have a superb ability to reproduce intricate patterns of color, shapes, and motion though dually possess extremely poor handwriting.

The inability to center written information on a page, in addition to deficits in sequencing letters and words in a straight line without tailing off, comes under the purview of constructional dyspraxia. Though faulty visual-spatial functioning certainly implicates right hemispheric functioning, poor spatial orientation skills can also occur due to a misallocation of attention resources due to the taxing demands of the writing process. After all, written language involves simultaneous memory skills for letter and word formations, spelling and syntactic rules, word retrieval and organization skills, and self-monitoring to ensure the desired goal of conveying meaning though print. Models of memory and attention such as Mirsky's (1999) have implicated the parietal lobes as being involved with the ability to focus attention on a specific cognitive task. Perhaps some students, especially younger ones who have little automaticity with respect to writing skills, simply cannot juggle all of the cognitive tasks and demands required to write a passage accurately. Since most of their cognitive energy becomes absorbed in the language aspect of writing, they can focus little attention on the mechanical output of written language production. Consequently, writing that tails off or seems excessively sloppy on a page may actually be due to fatigue stemming from an overworked attention system.

Lastly, it should be noted that the right hemisphere also has vastly different attention capacities from those of the left hemisphere, with damage to this region leading to unusual deficits Ramachandran (1998). For instance, the right hemisphere has a broad searchlight for attention that encompasses both the left and right visual fields. On the other hand, the left hemisphere has a much smaller searchlight confined to just the right visual field. Thus, damage to the left hemisphere generally does not lead to neglect since the right hemisphere can serve as a kind of attention *back-up* system. However, in most cases of damage to the right parietal lobe, there is hemi-neglect noted in the left-visual field only, as there are no back-up contingencies in the opposite hemisphere. Consequently, many stroke patients will demonstrate writing skills bunched toward the right side of the page, due to a general indifference to objects in the left visual field. In conclusion, neglect, difficulty with spatial constraints, poor centering skills, sloppy letter formations, and poor spacing between letters and words all come under the purview of constructional dyspraxia, a deficit due primarily to right hemispheric dysfunction.

# working memory and written language

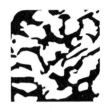

## Chapter 6

"Memory is the diary that we all carry with us."
— Oscar wilde

Ever wonder how a brilliant chess player can strategize hundreds of different spatial maneuvers to counter an opponent's pending tactics, or how a skilled comedian can instantly improvise a devilishly cunning retort to a would-be heckler? Better yet, how can some students master multiple-step mathematic equations without the need for paper and pencil calculation, or comprehend Macbeth upon an initial reading without the need for Cliff Notes? While most educators and psychologists would simply attribute these skilled attributes to intelligence, most cognitive neuropsychologists would argue that working memory is the underlying feature that allows for such higher-level mental functions. Clearly one of the most significant achievements of human mental evolution, is working memory which allows for the moment-to-moment awareness and instant retrieval of archived information (Goldman-Rakic, 1992). The ability to hold representational knowledge of our environment in mind, coupled with the mental flexibility to manipulate this knowledge in whatever manner we choose, is the essence of working memory.

As the "*blackboard of the mind,*" or what is sometimes called the "*cognitive workspace of our brain,*" working memory allows us to respond to tasks in a reflective manner as opposed to the reactive, reflex-oriented pursuits of other mammals. Hence, the concept of working memory is often viewed as the temporary storage of information to be used for a wide variety of cognitive tasks. Unlike periodic memory storage systems, where information is held for a set amount of time until consolidated or lost, working memory requires the instantaneous flow of information into conscious awareness to perform a given mental function. As Levine (1998) noted, short-term memory preserves information for a brief amount of time, while active working memory extends, modifies, or combines information with previously stored knowledge to perform a given cognitive task. In school, the ability to juggle multiple cognitive demands at once, such as listening and taking notes, reading and comprehending, and writing grammatically correct sentences to convey our thoughts, comes under the direct command of our working memory systems. There is no doubt that students with greater cognitive capacities for working memory possess a far greater ability to execute problem-solving tasks than students with limitations to their working memory systems, regardless of their overall intelligence.

Perhaps the concept of working memory and its critical importance to learning is best described by Baddeley's (2000) three-component system. According to Baddeley (2000), the first component of working memory is the *phonological loop* that holds and manipulates acoustic and speech-based information. It is assumed that auditory memory traces decay over a period of a few seconds, unless revived by rehearsing or replaying the information through our inner voice. This process - sometimes called subvocalization - is often an excellent strategy to assist students in developing an inner voice to support memory. The phonological loop presumably evolved for the purpose of speech production and storing phonemes in a meaningful manner, while more permanent linguistic representations were being constructed for long-term storage. For example, consider the average 5-year-old child who has already learned more than 2000 words and will learn up to 3000 more words in the upcoming school year alone (Baddeley, et. al., 1998). The task of forming long-term symbolic representations of the world based upon phonological storage is a key component of language acquisition. It is particularly suited to the retention of sound patterns in a sequential order, and can be easily measured by most digit span tasks (Baddeley, 2000). The phonological loop appears to be housed primarily in the left temporal lobes, as are most language processing areas.

The second component of working memory has been called the *visual-spatial sketchpad*, and presumably holds visual, spatial, and kinesthetic information in temporary storage in the form of mental imagery (Baddeley, 1998). This system remains a bit more complex than the phonological loop, with its rehearsal processes less clearly understood. However, the visual-spatial component of working memory seems to be more effective at storing a single complex pattern, but is not well suited for serial recall. Still, the ability to rely on visual imagery for the memorization of specific letter formations, spelling patterns, and punctuation rules, plays a vital role in the efficacy of written language production. The visual-spatial sketchpad appears to be housed primarily in the right hemisphere, along the inferior portions of the right parietal lobes and their interconnections with the temporal cortex (Baddeley, 2000). Figure 6-1 illustrates the neuroanatomical locations of both the visual-spatial sketchpad and the phonological loop.

## fIGURE 6-I

### components of working memory system

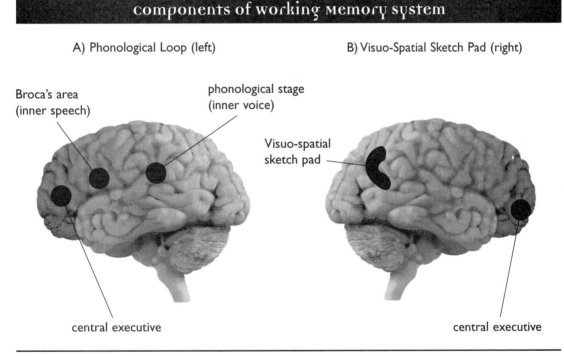

A) Phonological Loop (left)

B) Visuo-Spatial Sketch Pad (right)

Broca's area
(inner speech)

phonological stage
(inner voice)

Visuo-spatial
sketch pad

central executive

central executive

*Adapted from Carter, R., (1998). *Mapping the Mind.* Berkeley: University of California Press

The *central executive system* serves as the command post for controlling the functions of the two subsidiary or slave systems, the phonological rehearsal loop and the visual-spatial sketchpad. One of the primary purposes of the central executive system is to allocate attentional resources in a manner whereby two or more cognitive tasks can be performed in a simultaneous manner. The central executive control mechanism selectively attends to stimuli in sensory memory while simultaneously recycling both auditory and visual components until mediators are strategically employed to register them as a short-term memory. Throughout this process the central executive mechanism is probing into long-term storage in order to match the information with our previously stored knowledge base. Following the initial registration from sensory memory to short-term memory, there is a subsequent transfer to long-term memory for further consolidation and eventual retrieval. Figures 6-2 and 6-3 diagrams the essential components of this memory system.

## fIGURE 6-2

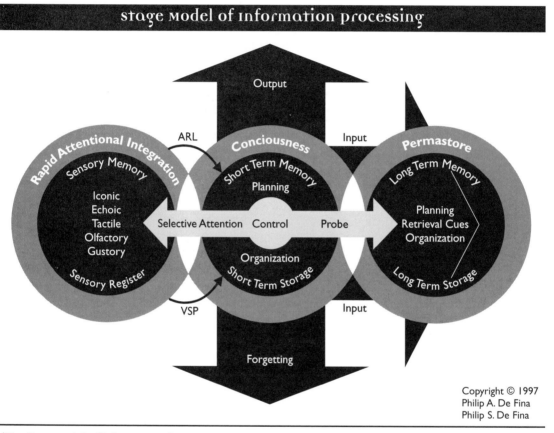

*De Fina model of Information Processing as a hybrid between Baddeley's model of "working memory" and the stage theory of memory processing (De Fina, 1997). Part I

This dynamic model of information processing can be conceptualized as three intermeshing wheels related to the essential components of working memory. In the center is the command and control mechanism of the supervisory attentional systems (SAS) of *central executive* (CE). This is where decision-making takes place as the brain selectively attends to sensory stimuli from the environment, while cross referencing it with information previously stored, by probing into long-term storage. Sensory memory (SM) is limited by the factor of time, usually milliseconds to seconds, and unless actively shifted to short-term storage by some form of mediator, it fades away or decays. Sensory storage is constantly bombarded by iconic, echoic, tactile, olfactory and gustatory information. Within milliseconds, rapid attentional integrations of these sensations impinge on our field of consciousness and a decision is made whether to sustain their attention while developing the appropriate strategy to assist with storage. A brief buffer delay assists with recycling this information while we simultaneously plan and organize efficient encoding strategies. Auditory-verbal information is recycled through the articulatory rehearsal loop (ARL) and visual-spatial information through the visual-spatial sketchpad (VSP). Pre-frontal neural networks within the lateral convexities of the frontal lobes assist in planning and organizing these strategies, so that the hippocampus can register the fragments of sensory stimuli into meaningful wholes. After this initial registration successfully occurs, there is a shift from short-term storage into that newly registered information can be reinforced. These newly formed memories are integrated and distributed neocortically by multiple neural networks into their appropriate electrochemical codes. These codes can be accessed like a hologram from one or more sensory retrieval mechanism at will. For instance, the olfactory sense of smell can identify an aroma as a pie baked by your grandmother. This one set of sensory data from a specific sensory modality can expand the repetoir of olfactory identification into other modalities which will assist in understanding the relevance of that particular sensory information. You may then revisualize your grandmother baking pies and may think about conversations you may have had while baking with her. The frontal lobes again play an important role with organization essential retreival cues for successful recall or recognition. Analysis and synthesis of information takes place in the posterior association cortex. Working memory occurs at all three phases simultaneously. Anterograde memory or acquisition of new knowledge is a tempero-limbic, cortical-subcortical phenomenon. The temporo-limbic system takes it from short term to long term storage, but this is monitored by prefrontal and posterior association areas. In long term storage, consolidation processes allow fusion of anterograde memory with information already in place - adding on to memory system. The supervisory attention system (SAS): lateral aspects of prefrontal cortex, integrated with amygdala and hippocampus monitor the cognitive and emotional relevance of the incoming sensory information so that it can be understood and utilized. Use of mediating strategies helps to categorize storage and retrieval. Remember this is an active, dynamic process.

## fIGURE 6-3

### stage model of information processing

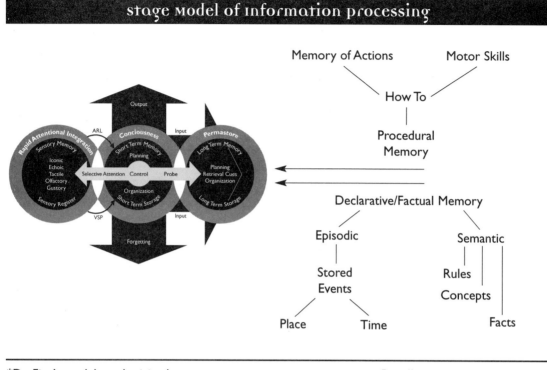

*De Fina's model emphasizing long term memory storage components. Part II

In addition, the central executive system allows for the reflection on and critical analysis of incoming information, so long as the two slave systems can work together keeping the information alive in conscious awareness. From an evolutionary standpoint, the ability to select the most appropriate information from the immediate environment and maintain it actively until the necessary planning of action has been completed has profound survival implications (Baddeley, 1998). For instance, the central executive system is housed in the prefrontal cortex, an area that marked a critical leap in human evolution. Approximately one and a half million years ago, the frontal lobes of the brain expanded by about 40 percent, to create large areas of new gray matter that formed the prefrontal cortex (Carter, 1998). This development can be seen in fossil fragments that show the bones of the skull protruding outward, thus creating a high, flat forehead similar to the shape of a modern-day skull. It stands to reason that this expansion of neocortical development enabled higher-level, increasingly sophisticated learning to commence. Consequently, human beings broke away from their mammalian counterparts by developing skills such as abstract thinking, critical analysis, and symbolic representation of linguistic concepts. An often-overlooked feature of prefrontal lobe development was the unique ability of human beings to hold representations of the physical world in the mind's eye, even when those objects were no longer present. These cognitive phenomena are components of the working memory system. Jean Piaget noted that infants 8 months of age or younger have no conceptual grasp of object permanence. Thus, if distracted after being shown a toy inside a box, an infant does not have the capacity to recall that the toy is still present, despite being inside the box. In other words, out-of-sight literally means out-of-mind. Therefore, the ability to develop object permanence simply reflects the emergence of working memory coming to fruition in the developing prefrontal cortex, in order to store representations of the outside world when these objects are no longer in view. (It is important to note that the prefrontal cortex receives sensory information through the dorsomedial (DMN) of the thalamus. So, we can further define the anterior tertiary zone or prefrontal cortex as the recipient of sensory information transferred from the DMN of the thalamus.)

The cognitive evolution of working memory resulted in people in being able to respond to their environment in a reflexive fashion, based on emotion no longer existed. Notwithstanding, the expansion and subsequent development of the prefrontal cortex allowed information to be stored and reflected upon, and therefore triggered a sense of reason and purpose coupled with rational decision-making. Hence, working memory is closely linked to the critical role that the frontal lobes play in the temporal organization of behavior and in controlling the proper sequence in which mental operations are deployed when engaged in a cognitive task (Goldberg, 2001). As will be discussed in the following chapter, the central executive system plays a crucial role in the efficacy with which students engage in virtually any cognitive task, especially written language. Table 6-1 lists some of the major academic pitfalls of faulty working memory systems for students.

## TABLE 6-1

### Academic pitfalls of working memory dysfunctions

1. **MATH:** Tendency to lose one's place in the middle of solving a mathematic equation. In the process of performing one computation, a student forgets what to do next.

2. **READING:** Difficulty with comprehension and remembering the information from the top of a page while reading the final paragraph.

3. **WRITING:** Problems recalling the simultaneous skills needed for effective written production. This includes difficulty remembering spelling, punctuation, spacing, and organization and clarity principles while writing.

4. **LISTENING:** Confusion and comprehension problems during extended explanations or multiple step instructions.

5. **SPEAKING:** A tendency for a student to raise their hand only to forget what they were going to say, or lose their train of thought while speaking. Some word finding issues and tip-of-the tongue phenomena might be present as well.

6. **ATTENTION:** A tendency for more immediate needs and gratifications to undermine more long term goals. For instance, a student may leave their seat to sharpen a pencil, only to become more engaged by a peer, then forget the original intention of leaving their seat.

*Adapted from Levine, M.D., & Reed, M., (1999) Developmental variation and learning disorders. Massachusetts: Educators Publishing Services, Inc. (p.75).

Perhaps more than any other academic skill, written language represents the final common pathway in which multiple psychological constructs can converge. The ability of working memory to recall spelling rules, sentence structures, variations of punctuation, and syntax, simultaneously, as a student attempts to organize a specific thought, remains critically important. Consequently, the inability of the central executive system component of working memory to allocate the necessary attentional resources to each of these individual pursuits poses an immense threat to effective written language production. Perhaps this is why students with attention deficit disorder have more difficulty with written language than with virtually any other academic endeavor. For instance, in a study by Resta and Eliot (1994), it was found that students with attention deficit disorder were at a distinct disadvantage in successfully mastering both written language and copying skills. Essentially, children with attention deficits are hampered by problems of distractibility, which subsequently leads to deficits in working memory producing disastrous effects on written production. They cannot simultaneously process what they want to say and actually carry our the process of writing it.

A common complaint among teachers and parents is that some students can express an answer verbally, but remain unable to deliver the same response in written form. The true culprit may lie in a faulty working memory system that prevents a student from juggling all of the necessary sub-processes required for written output. In other words, the cognitive workspace necessary to perform the written task is just too small, and/or inefficient, and as a result, then some element of written production must be dismissed. For some students, the daunting task of beginning such an endeavor will be so overwhelming that they have tremendous difficulty getting started on the assignment, thereby requiring extra teacher assistance. These students may have little difficulty beginning an assignment, while others complete the task in a hurried fashion, with much sloppiness noted. In essence, the attentional resources are allocated toward the linguistic end of production at the expense of self-monitoring graphomotor output. According to Annoni et. al., (1998), the degree to which a written language task has been *"automated"* also plays a key role in the deployment of attention resources. In other words, poorly learned or less automated types of tasks require more attention than tasks that are more routinely executed. Hence, a student with outstanding writing fluency and problematic spelling needs to dedicate more cognitive energy, namely attention, toward the less skilled task of spelling, in order to produce a legible written language product. In conclusion, working memory is the cognitive construct that allows for the mental gymnastics required to synthesize and bind the vast array of linguistic and motor skills necessary to produce the complex task of written language production.

In essence, new learning or anterograde memory is often synonymous with the concept of working memory, and relies on a number of similar underlying systems dependent upon multiple anatomic sites with specific electrochemical environments. The encoding of new memories and the retrieval (recall or recognition) of previously stored information utilizes components of the same neural pathways. Therefore, it becomes problematic to separate the processes of initial remembering from retrieving. Modality specific retrieval mechanisms are activated by visual, auditory or tactile-kinesthetic routes depending upon the task at hand. For instance, when copying written information from the external environment, students rely upon certain visual pathways and mechanisms. When internally accessing information for spontaneous written expression, the same components and pathways also become activated to re-visualize letters and words, and then become organized into specific motor sequences for precise writing. According to Calvin (1996), the contents of our thoughts are extracted from embedded spatio-temporal themes activated by retrieval mechanisms, which are driven by certain chemical codes. While there is no one area of the brain responsible for the complexities of memory processing, per se, the driving force behind efficient memory and retrieval processes emanates from subcortical limbic and basal ganglia structures. The left hippocampal formation is responsible for pulling together dispersed verbal components of cortical sensory information traveling from the left posterior tertiary zone (temporal-parietal-occipital cortex) to these subcortical regions. The initial registration of the cognitive aspects of semantic-linguistic processing is a left hippocampal-entorhinal cortical (tempero-limbic) phenomenon, and the emotional components are processed through the contiguous interconnected region of the amygdala. The visual-spatial aspects of non-verbal registration are processed from dispersed sensory information in the right posterior tertiary zone to the right hippocampal and amygdalofugal pathways. Further consolidation continues after this initial registration, both of which are directed by prefrontal cortical structures within the aforementioned anterior tertiary zone.

According to Damasio (1994), these so-called covergence zones are responsible for integrating memory components during the retrieval process. Within milliseconds to seconds, hundreds of words can be organized into their appropriate linguistic-semantic order, and motorically converted to speech sounds or transcribed into a written language format. In fact, Kandel et. al., (1999), isolated the protein molecule CREB that initiates the process of storage in both short and long term memories. Therefore, memory can be viewed upon as a mathematical probability that neurons will fire in a predetermined pattern, which is influenced by specific neurotansmitter substances in the frontal-temporal-subcortical circuits of the brain. Excitatory or inhibitory pathways that allow for the expression of these memories differentially modulate each circuit directly or indirectly.

Verbally mediated learning disabilities often times impact on the linguistic-semantic aspects of writing which usually involve a high degree of working memory impairment. The details of episodic memories for events, as well as associative aspects of verbal memories, are slowly processed in learning disabled children very slowly. These children have random and poorly organized search strategies which result in slow and diminished retrieval, due primarily to their inefficient use of retrieval cues during fluency tasks. The systematic search for the appropriate exemplars within specific categories of words are both qualitatively and quantitatively impaired. The uptake and ulitization of glucose metabolic activity and the generation of corresponding electromagnetic fields may be compromised as well in these individuals. Memory and *"executive"* functions are usually the most sensitive indices of neurocognitive dysfunction. In children with specific learning disabilities, there is a high degree of co-morbidity with various forms of attention and memory deficits. It is extremely important to evaluate these functions as part of the routine assessment of children with reading, written language and math disabilities.

Many of the well-standardized memory batteries for children are suitable for assessing the underlying strengths and weaknesses in acquisition and retrieval of new information. Distracting techniques such as the Peterson-Peterson paradigm and the selective and restrictive reminders of the Buschke-Fuld techniques (1974), can be valuable in separating out acquisition from retrieval. This has both neuroanatomical and physiological implications, and is extremely useful in developing a student's Individualized Educational Program (IEP). For example, in a study conducted by Fedio & Mirsky (1969), children with lateralized seizure foci were evaluated for both verbal and non-verbal memories. While short-term memory was relatively unimpaired, a 5-minute delayed recall task demonstrated significant impairment in children with right hemisphere lesions who also did poorly on non-verbal and visual spatial aspects of memory. Children with left hemisphere impairment had more problems with verbal recall. Furthermore, there is plenty of evidence demonstrating specific memory deficits associated with Traumatic Brain Injury (TBI) as well. Children who sustain a mechanical injury to the brain can develop an acquired reading and written language disorder with associated *"dysexecutive"* functioning and memory deficits. It is extremely important to assess these neurocognitive functions and the specific course of recovery when these children or adolescents re-enter school.

Interventions for memory impairment need to be specifically developed based upon the nature and extent of the disability. There are many memory-enhancing techniques such as rehearsal, mnemonics, imaging, etc. These techniques must be carefully selected depending upon the neuropsychological strengths and weaknesses that emerge from the evaluation. Interventions should not be applied as a shotgun approach, but rather should be tailored to the specific needs of the child. Unfortunately many IEP goals tend to be arbitrarily selected from a menu of potential interventions, and then simply cut and pasted into the report. Prior to developing appropriate interventions, the diagnostician should understand the type of memory impairment (e.g., semantic, episodic, rote, procedural, automatic etc.) and the modality in which the impairment exists (e.g., visual, auditory, tactile, etc.). Table 6-2 illustrates a list of commonly used memory strategies often used in school systems.

## TABLE 6-2

| commonly used memory strategies | | |
|---|---|---|
| rehearsal/repetition | outlining | put to music |
| association | role-playing | game designs |
| chunking/clustering | paraphrasing | mind mapping |
| categorizing | peer teaching | discussing |
| imaging/visual aids | summarizing | drawing/artwork |
| mnemonic-devices | time lines | contextualizing |
| graphic organizers | rhyming | emotional charging |
| semantic strategies | acronyms | sorting |
| humor/exaggeration | color coding | physical reinforcement |

As a general rule, students who are taught something new need to have it frequently reinforced over time. The reinforcement schedule should be on the same day, within 48 hours of the intial learning trials, and up to a week or two after the initial learning exposure. By minimizing interference and promoting active reasoning, students can emphasize what is important to remember, and can actively think about this new information for a greater depth of processing. When encoding new memories, students transform information into a format compatible for eventual use in long term storage (LTS). The most salient aspects of the stimuli are attended to in order to make sense of incoming data, while simultaneously cross-referencing it with data previously stored. When memory deficits arise, the information may fail to reach LTS even if properly organized for registration. After successful initial registration, the information must be maintained and eventually consolidated into long-term storage.

When working with children it is important to understand the developmental limitations of memory processing. In fact, most students use various mediators or strategies (e.g., rehearsal, chunking, clustering, mnemonic association, imagery, etc.) in order to assist in transferring information from short-term storage (STS) to LTS. Both the qualitative and quantitative efficiency of these mediators tend to change with age. For instance, just 10% of five-year olds use rehearsal strategies; however, the same method is used by approximately 60% of seven-year olds and 85% of ten-year olds (Gaddes and Edgell, 1994). Though five-year olds produce greater recall in visual memory, greater recognition does not consistently occur until approximately age ten, due to better rehearsal strategies. Five to six-year olds do not use category-based learning strategies, but rather rely on rote rehearsal and/or association. Although younger children (4-5) can utilize categories, they fail to initiate categorical organization. These younger children usually link items in terms of functional categories (e.g., cake-fork), or by shape or form characteristics. Older children (7-9) can do better at learning to organize conceptual categories (e.g., food-plate). Free recall improves with age across categories due to maturation of the frontal "executive" system and its connections to the temporal-limbic system. Clustering and categorical learning increases in efficiency as the brain matures. Older children incorporate relevant information from previously rehearsed trials into subsequent rehearsals. These children use a single retrieval cue or target stimulus to recall multiple components that need to be remembered, hence, quicker and more accurate remembering. Toddlers (3-4) cannot accurately form memories of episodes since their neural apparatus is so immature, which disallows them from extracting relevant memories from earlier experiences. Therefore, as retrieval cue usage becomes more efficient, memories then become recalled more easily and accurately (Gaddes & Edgell, 1994)

In summary, children with learning disabilities need more time to effectively carry out memory searches while probing into long-term storage. The neuropsychological profile of these children often reveal slower and inefficient processing when transferring information from STS into LTS. As a result, organizational and planning strategies are often deficient in this clinical group as well. Poor processing of phonological codes along with less efficient use of rehearsal strategies and retrieval cues are noteworthy. Since most brain dysfunction has associated memory impairment and dysexecutive functioning, the neuropsychological profiles of these students are useful in understanding the nature and degree of memory impairment. Therefore, when training students with specific use of mnemonic strategies, teachers should take into consideration the relative strengths and weaknesses of a student's neuropsychological profile. This will lead to more independent and consistent memory enhancing abilities. After all, when students are taught strategies commensurate with their ability level, they tend to become more successful learners. The psychologist can assist in developing appropriate interventions for the educator by comprehensibly assessing and reporting the relevant cognitive functions that underly these processes. The qualitative data that is observed during the evaluation process (how the student gets to the right or wrong answers) are invaluable elements that need to be incorporated into the intervention plan. This utilization of data from a process viewpoint is what makes the evaluation worthwhile for the educator.

| Steven G. Feifer, Ed.S., NCSP    Philip A. De Fina, Ph.D., ABPdN

# executive functions and written language

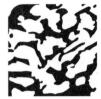

## Chapter 7

*"for I am a bear of very little brain and long words bother me."*
— winnie the pooh

All professions, particularly the more scientifically oriented ones, have certain phrases that encapsulate the espirit de corps of their discipline as it makes its ascent toward popular culture. For instance, the *human genome project* has engulfed the science of molecular biology, *deductions* serves as the buzz word in tax accounting, *Dow Jones* sets the boundaries for would-be Wall Street investors, and *attention deficit disorder* has dominated the diagnostic landscape of psychology and pediatric medicine. Additionally, certain scientific disciplines have endured their own complement of faulty pseudo-science. Chemists still have alchemy, physicists have cold fusion, astronomy continues to deal with astrology, and psychology has psychoanalysis (Sagan, 1996). For the last two decades, one of the most prevalent and now almost fashionable types of mental health conditions manifested in our society remains attention deficit disorder. In fact, it seems that both educators and mental health practitioners view any deviation from the norm with respect to school performance, social relationships, or vocational aptitude as stemming in part from attention deficit disorder. It is viewed as a distinct entity, somewhat like the common cold, as those who struggle to maintain their concentration or need some explanation for failure wonder whether *"I have it or I don't."* The taxonomy of such a simplistic classification system speaks volumes for our continuing insistence on explaining the world's phenomena through the invention of artificial categories, much as our ancestors attempted to comprehend their surroundings by fabricating a separate deity for each event.

It is seductively tempting to explain behavioral deficiencies using a categorical model, whether spawned from reality or fabrication, which precisely defines the reason for ineptness in a given pursuit. Unfortunately, as these notions pervade widely held belief systems and garner mass appeal from religious, political, and even some academic institutions, it becomes increasingly difficult to redirect human thinking toward a more scientific paradigm for these events. After all, most behavioral traits do not arise from a simple cause-and-effect or linear type of attribution model, but rather stem from an amalgam of conditions and functions, more modular in nature and depicted in shades or degrees of behavioral manifestations. Fortunately, psychology has leaned on neuropsychology, which in turn has leaned on the technological advances from the medical sciences, to forge a more comprehensive means of conceptualizing multiple traits. With respect to inattention, neuropsychology has coined a new buzz word for the 21st century that describes clusters of inattentive behavior and faulty decision making skills: namely, *executive functioning*.

Since neuropsychology is the study of interactions between brain functions and behavior, it is a particularly informative discipline with respect to written language. Perhaps no other academic pursuit demands a higher order of executive functioning than written expression. The mere act of writing requires a certain amount of self-regulation in order to direct the complicated and interrelated capacities of thought, processing, and production. High levels of executive functioning are especially important for skilled writing because it is an intentional task that is often self-planned and self-sustained (Zimmerman & Riesemberg, 1997). As noted previously, writing is a difficult endeavor for a variety of reasons, as the demands of transcription require both motor and cognitive resources. For example, writing requires planning, sentence generation, and revision skills orchestrated in a manner to allow the writer to switch attention seamlessly between these functions. The phrase *executive functioning* has been used in the neuropsychological literature to denote several aspects of independent, purposeful, and self-regulating behavior (Lezak, 1995). According to Scardamalia & Bereiter (1986), executive functioning enhances written language performance by providing the building blocks or subroutines used in planning and executing a task. In addition, by developing and rehearsing a subroutine such as planning, monitoring, evaluating, and revising a task, the beginning writer can now make strategic adjustments with much greater precision and more self-assurance. Consequently, the more success a student experiences with written language, the greater the intrinsic motivation to become even more accomplished at this task.

In essence, these assumptions about executive control and writing suggest that skilled writers generally have more executive control than less skilled writers. Given developmental theories such as those proposed by Piaget, it is not surprising that executive functioning improves for developing writers with age and education. Though individual differences in the executive control functions predict individual differences in writing, learning strategies related to executive functioning can enhance the performance of developing writers. Table 7-1 lists the salient features of executive functioning with respect to their contribution to the written language process.

## TABLE 7-1

### salient features of executive functioning and written language

| EXECUTIVE FUNCTION | WRITING FEATURE |
|---|---|
| 1. **Initiating:** Difficulty beginning a written language activity. | • Poor idea generation<br>• Often unfocused<br>• Poor independent learner |
| 2. **Sustaining:** Difficulty persisting on assignment. | • Lose track of thoughts<br>• Can begin activity, though has difficulty finishing activity<br>• Sentences disjointed and meaning is disorganized |
| 3. **Inhibiting:** Difficulty stopping a thought on paper. | • Impulsive<br>• Distractible<br>• Fidgety and restless while writing<br>• Additions to words when spelling, such as "streeet" |
| 4. **Shifting:** Difficulty switching topics in print. | • Perseverations<br>• Stuck on one topic throughout passage<br>• Upset by changes in routine when writing about multiple events<br>• Poor writing from dictation |
| 5. **Organizing:** Difficulty organizing information in a particular writing framework. | • Frequent erasers<br>• Forget the main idea<br>• Messy desk and workspace<br>• Disjointed content with poor transitions between sentences |
| 6. **Planning:** Difficulty forecasting a set of circumstances or events. | • Poor verbal fluency<br>• Incorrect spacing of words and letters<br>• Cohesive ties lacking between sentences<br>• Poor use of lines on paper when forming words |

| | |
|---|---|
| **7. Self-Monitoring:** Difficulty recognizing strengths and weaknesses in writing language | Unaware of spelling miscues<br>• Unaware of faulty punctuation or incorrect grammar and usage<br>• Believe work is good despite contrary evidence<br>• Sloppy handwriting<br>• Careless errors/Limited |

Graham and Harris (2000) cite numerous studies indicating that proficient writers spend more time planning and focusing their attention on text-level concerns and making revisions and are more knowledgeable about processes of executive control than less skilled writers. In fact, their research has demonstrated that overall written language performance for beginning writers can indeed improve with direct instruction in executive processing. Some studies indicate that improvements result from instruction in the use of just a single self-regulatory strategy such as goal setting behaviors (Graham, et. al., 1995; Page-Voth & Graham, 1999). However, other studies have suggested that improvements in written language were associated with multiple self-regulatory procedures (Sawyer, et. al., 1992). In fact, a recent study by De La Paz (1999) illustrated the benefit of instruction in multiple components of executive functioning to improve writing performance. During a 4-week period, middle school teachers taught seventh and eighth grade students to use a self-regulation heuristic to guide their essay writing. The heuristic contained several strategies for advanced and continuous planning, such as goal setting, seeking information, organizing, and self-monitoring. The results indicated that overall written language performance showed marked improvements among all students. Therefore, it would appear that teaching an array of strategies aimed at increased executive control improves written language performance. Chapter 10 discusses specific remediation strategies geared toward enhanced planning and self-regulatory behaviors in the written language process.

Without question, the development of writing competence depends on high levels of executive functioning. In fact, there tends to be much more literature and data on the role of executive function in writing than there is on the impact of basic transcription skills such as handwriting and spelling. However, mastery of transcription skills are extremely important because these skills initially require and demand considerable attentional resources. Until a child is fluent in the mechanics of writing, there will be continued difficulty on the *higher-level* components of written language, as those students who struggle with handwriting and spelling allocate too much of their attentional resources for these lower-level skills. Consequently, there are few cognitive resources left to attend to the complex task of organizing and developing their thoughts and ideas on paper. This process taxes active working memory and interferes with higher-order skills such as planning and content generation (Graham, 1990). In fact, young writers find transcription skills so demanding that they minimize the use of other writing processes, such as planning and revision, due to the attention resources being deployed (McCutchen, 1996). Arrested writing development is in part attributable to difficulty with transcription skills when the burden is so great that it causes children to avoid writing and develop a negative self-perception regarding the written language process.

There is increasing evidence that writing competence depends both on high levels of executive control and mastery of basic transcription skills. For instance, in a study by Berninger et. al. (1997), first grade students at risk for handwriting difficulties were randomly assigned to five handwriting treatment groups, while others were assigned to phonological awareness training to improve their writing skills. The written language performance improved most for those students with explicit training in handwriting skills. A study by Jones and Christiensen (1999) found that instruction aimed at improving the letter formation and handwriting fluency skills of first-grade children with poor handwriting enhanced story-writing performance. Finally, a follow-up study by Berninger et. al. (1998) indicated that spelling instruction that emphasized the learning of common phoneme-spelling associations and used spelling words when writing a short composition resulted in improvements in spelling as well as increased word production. In summary, it would appear that more skilled writers demonstrated greater mastery of transcription skills than less skilled writers, that transcription skills improve with age and education, and that individual differences in transcription skills predict writing achievement. Furthermore, deficits with transcription skills force children to allocate greater attention resources, leaving few executive controls left to monitor the written production process. Hence, faulty executive control processes can both directly and indirectly result in writing difficulties.

It should be noted that some children have difficulty with transcription skills due to motor impairments of the small muscle groups needed for fluent letter formation on paper. Graphomotor dysfunctions may indicate gaps or breakdowns in the connections between the brain and hand. These dysfunctions take the form of generalized fine-motor deficiencies, such that drawing, tracing, using scissors, and writing pose difficulties. There are many students who demonstrate exclusive graphomotor dysfunction, meaning that their fine motor problems affect only their written language skills. These children may have a high aptitude for art or mechanics, despite their writing being slow, laborious, and sometimes illegible. Table 7-2 illustrates three common forms of graphomotor dysfunctions.

## TABLE 7-2

| Three forms of Graphomotor Dysfunctions | |
|---|---|
| DYSFUNCTION | WRITING DEFICIT |
| Motor Memory Dysfunctions | • Poor motor output and production.<br>• Unable to recall sequences of muscle movements needed to produce letters.<br>• Difficulty recalling letter shapes.<br>  Writing is slow, hesitant, and labored.<br>• Inconsistent letter formations.<br>• Frequent reversals, erasers, and reduced legibility.<br>• Prefer printing to cursive due to fewer motor sequences. |
| Graphomotor Production Deficits | • Poor coordination and unstable pencil grip.<br>• Slower paced writing.<br>• Writing dominated by larger muscles of wrist and forearm.<br>• History of speech articulation difficulty often present.<br>• Inconsistent writing pressure.<br>• Muscle fatigue. |
| Motor Feedback Deficits | • Eyes close to monitor the pencil visually.<br>• Inability to monitor writing instrument as reported by small nerve endings in joints of fingers. |

*Adapted from Levine, M.D., & Reed, M., (1999). *Developmental Variation and Learning Disorders.*
Massachusetts: Educators Publishing Service, Inc.

Executive functions appear to have a generalized neuroanatomical base housed within the prefrontal cortex. This brain region accounts for approximately 29% of the total cortex in humans, 17% in the chimpanzee, 11.5% in the gibbon, 7% in the dog, and just 3.5% in the cat (Goldberg, 2001). A unique feature of the prefrontal cortex is that it directly interconnects with every distinct functional unit of the brain. Hence, damage to prefrontal regions tends to produce more global and widespread disturbances, as opposed to more specific cognitive deficits. According to Goldberg (2001), executive functioning generally refers to the brain's capacity to execute the following six steps in order to accomplish virtually any problem-solving task:

## TABLE 7-3

### six steps for every purposeful Behavior

1. The behavior must be initiated in some capacity.
2. A goal of action must be formulated.
3. A plan of action to execute the desired goal must be forged.
4. The means by which the plan can be accomplished must be selected.
5. The various steps of the plan must be executed in their proper sequential order.
6. A comparison must be made between the objective and outcome of action.

* Adapted from Goldberg, E., (2001). The executive brain: Frontal lobes and the civilized mind. New York: Oxford University Press. (p.116).

The prefrontal cortex is comprised of three main areas, each of which play a vital role in the modulation of attention to achieve a purposeful goal. The **dorsolateral circuit,** whose primary projections go through the basal ganglia, helps to organize a behavioral response to solve complex problem-solving tasks (Chow & Cummings, 1999). In essence, there is an actual brain region responsible for getting us out of bed in the morning, planning our day, and balancing the duties of how much time to allocate for homework versus baseball practice versus completing household chores. In fact, damage to the dorsolateral cortex produces an almost *"pseudo-depressive"* state in which an inability to initiate behavior is present along with an indifference to virtually any endeavor or activity. In its extreme form, damage to the dorsolateral cortex can even produce an indifference to pain (Goldberg, 2001). While behavior modification has been a popular intervention technique with students who are unmotivated or indifferent to academic outcomes, this type of intervention would clearly have no impact on a student with faulty dorsolateral functioning. There simply is no interest or desire to achieve a positive outcome, no matter the consequence. With respect to written language and paper and pencil tasks, the behaviors outlined in Table 7-4 may also be present.

## TABLE 7-4

### Executive Functioning Deficits with Disorders of the Dorsolateral Cortex

| classification | impaired functions |
| --- | --- |
| Poor organizational strategies | • Segmented drawing<br>• Poor organization of material<br>• Poor word list generation<br>• Reduced design fluency<br>• Poor planning<br>• Difficulty initiating tasks |
| Poor memory search strategies | • Poor recall of remote information<br>• Poor recall of new information<br>• Poor idea generation |
| Poor cognitive set shifting | • Inability to use verbal skills to guide thought process<br>• Tendency to perseverate on topics<br>• Poor concept development and lack of insight<br>• Difficulty prioritizing salient information<br>• Poor sequential motor skills |

* Adapted from Chow, T.W., & Cummings, J.L., (1999). Frontal-subcortical circuits. In B.L. Miller & J.L. Cummings, *The human frontal lobes: functions and disorder,* (p. 5), New York: Guilford Publications.

The second region of the prefrontal cortex that comprises the more generic realm of behaviors known as executive functions is the ***orbitofrontal cortex***. The orbitofrontal cortex mediates empathic, civil, and socially appropriate behavior, with acute personality change being the hallmark feature of orbitofrontal dysfunction (Chow & Cummings, 1999). In other words, students who have difficulty empathizing with the feelings of others, demonstrating poor judgment, having awkward social skills, and manifesting extreme impulsivity and/or obsessive-like behaviors may have deficits in this brain region. Often, these students are tagged with having an attention deficit disorder when in actuality the central problem is poor self-regulation. Unlike deficits with dorsolateral regions, cognitive problem solving skills often remain intact. While serotonin is one of the main neurotransmitters that help modulate the dorsolateral cortex, dopamine weighs heavily on the orbitofrontal cortex, especially in the left hemisphere.

There are devastating academic consequences associated with orbitofrontal dysfunction, despite the fact that general intelligence scores remain fundamentally intact. This is due in part to an inability to self-monitor academic work, a tendency to make careless errors, and poor time-management skills. These types of errors more often reveal themselves in the context of classroom learning situations as opposed to individual testing and evaluation procedures. One reason examiners often overlook this particular component of executive functioning is that examiners serve as the *executive functions* for students during the testing procedure. In other words, by monitoring time, repeating directions, and basically instructing a student of what to do and when to do it, the examiner serves as sort of a pseudo-orbitofrontal cortex during the evaluation. With respect to written language, the ability to self-monitor written work may be the most critical feature of accomplished writing. The passage must be constantly monitored to determine if the piece is suitable for the intended audience, if the tone and language are appropriate, and if it conforms to the structural requirements of a letter, essay, resume, etc. The ability to review work to garner feedback is essential for students to monitor their own effectiveness as communicators and evaluate their own skill level in meeting the goals of an assignment.

It should be noted that these same attributes are vital for successful social skill functioning as well, as students constantly need to self-monitor the extent to which their own behavior is in accord with the demands of a specific environmental context. Therefore, poor self-monitoring is also a core dysfunction of students with attention deficit disorder, as these students tend to have rather poor social skill functioning. Consequently, they may laugh in inappropriate situations, use an aggressive tone of voice unknowingly, and state critical remarks when trying to engage peers, due to an inability to monitor their own emotional state based upon feedback from a given social situation. Table 7-5 lists some of the behavioral deficits observed with students who have deficits in their orbitofrontal cortex.

## TABLE 7-5

| Executive Functioning Deficits with Disorders of the Orbitofrontal Cortex | |
|---|---|
| classification | impaired functions |
| Personality changes | • Poor regulation of emotions<br>• Irritability<br>• Poor tactfulness<br>• Antisocial behavior<br>• Extreme impulsivity<br>• Inability to self-monitor |
| Mood disorders | • Depression<br>• Mania<br>• Rigidity in thinking patterns |
| Poor environmental learning | • Inappropriate emotional responses in normal situations<br>• Poor stimulus – response learning<br>• Difficulty with transitions<br>• Difficulty changing cognitive sets<br>• Difficulty recognizing reinforcing stimuli |

* Adapted from Chow, T.W., & Cummings, J.L., (1999). Frontal-subcortical circuits. In B.L. Miller & J.L. Cummings: *The human frontal lobes: functions and disorder,* (p. 7), New York: Guilford Publications.

The third region of the prefrontal cortex that plays a vital role in the vast array of behavior functions that comprise the executive functions is the ***anterior cingulate cortex***. The anterior cingulate cortex supplies a multitude of functions linking attention capabilities with that of a given cognitive task. According to Carter (1998), this region helps the brain divert its conscious energies either toward internal cognitive events or external incoming stimuli. In fact, the anterior cingulate cortex has been found to be under-active (i.e. a hypofrontality with regard to glucose metabolic activity), in schizophrenic patients, thus explaining some of their difficulty separating their own thoughts from outside voices (Carter, 1998). Furthermore, the anterior cingulate cortex also functions to allow us both to feel and interpret emotions. Significant impairment to this brain region can produce a wide variety of peculiar emotional responses, most of which seem related to an inability to appreciate emotions. Apathy, akinetic mutism, reduced creative thought, and poor response inhibition are just a few of the behavioral characteristics modulated by the anterior cingulate cortex (Chow &

Cummings, 1999).

With respect to written language, the inability to modulate attention effectively to the multitude of symbolic rules and representations needed for effective writing seems to be the hallmark feature of faulty anterior cingulate functioning. There is a great deal of evidence suggesting that the anterior cingulate cortex plays a vital though often overlooked role in the ability to make word associations (Posner & Raichle, 1994). In other words, skilled writing ultimately comes down to the proficiency with which a student can carefully select from among the 80,000 words in the English language a given word or phrase that best connotes a particular thought, idea, or explanation. Most words are housed in semantic categories, thus facilitating instantaneous access and retrieval. For instance, the word *"change"* as a form of money also activates related words such as *"penny"*, *"nickel"*, and *"dime"*. In doing so, the writer has various options from which to choose under the semantic category of *change*, as various related words also come to mind. However, the word *change* also has another meaning, and can be used to connote an alternative or different way of doing things. This secondary meaning must be suppressed in order for the monetary meaning of change to be more readily available to our thinking process (Posner & Raichle, 1994). Therefore, the anterior cingulate gyrus must not only focus our attention inward toward a given semantic category, but also must inhibit conflicting semantic categories in order to maximize vigilance on a particular topic area.

One extreme symptom noted with damage to this brain area is akinetic mutism, or lack of drive or initiative. In other words, nothing comes to mind in these individuals due to the inability of the anterior cingulate cortex to exercise control over the attention process as it pertains to directing our thoughts in a goal-directed pursuit. In summary, the anterior cingulate cortex functions to draw our attention to internally represented ideas and thoughts while simultaneously inhibiting conflicting ideas and thoughts in order for information to enter working memory. It stands to reason that proficient writers have the innate capacity to retrieve multiple words under a given topic area (anterior cingulate cortex) and draw these words into working memory or what is called our cognitive workspace for further reflection and enhancement before delivering a cogent response on paper. Students with attention deficit disorder are severely restricted in the writing process as the attention mechanisms under the control of the anterior cingulate cortex may be impaired, thereby, resulting in conflicting word recall as well as reduced working memory skills.

## FIGURE 7-1

**Attentional Mechanisms in the Brain**

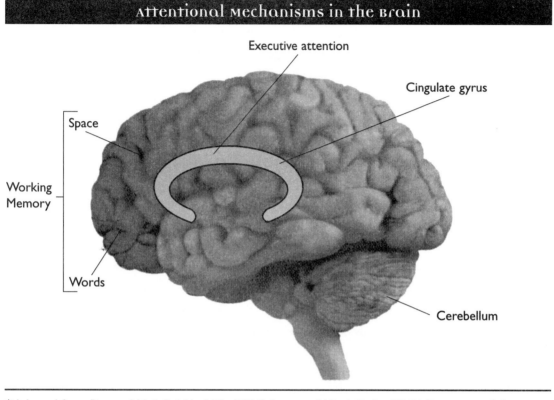

Executive attention

Cingulate gyrus

Space

Working
Memory

Words

Cerebellum

---

* Adapted from Posner, M.I. & Raichle, M.E., (1994). Images of Mind. Oxford: W.H. Freeman and Company.

---

The three major divisions of the frontal lobes differ in function, though each is intricately involved with behavioral output. For instance, the most posterior division, which lies in the first two ridges of the central sulcus, is the *precentral cortex*. This is the primary motor cortex that mediates overall movement (though not isolated muscles). This area of the brain also has important connections with the *cerebellum, basal ganglia,* and the motor division of the *thalamus,* with damage resulting in weakness or paralysis of the corresponding body part. The *premotor cortex* is just anterior to the pre-central area, and is a site primarily responsible for the integration of motor skills and learned action sequences. This area directly relates to writing behavior with damage resulting in the disruption of the motor components of complex acts, producing discontinuous or uncoordinated movements and impaired motor skills, coupled with reduced limb strength as well. The *supplemental motor area* mediates preparatory arousal to action at a preconscious stage in the generation of movement, with damage resulting in the disruption of motor initiation (ideomotor apraxia). The ability to copy rapidly executed hand movements may be associated with damage to this area as well. Lastly, the *supplemental motor area* contains those mechanisms involved in the initiation and programming of fine hand movements, with deficits resulting in more severe forms of dysgraphia.

In summary, since writing demands the highest form of cognitive processing, the integration of brain and motor functions is essential for proper written language development. Damage or dysfunction to the frontal lobes can severely disturb executive functioning processes that control integration of brain functions and consequently disrupt the ability to write. Fortunately, certain aspects of the executive functioning domain can be taught, enabling writers to approach problems in an orderly rather than a chaotic manner. Teaching self-regulation strategies is usually successful because it provides internal cures to students who do not often spontaneously generate strategies while learning novel tasks. Once a student learns selection and self-monitoring skills, control is gained in areas previously directed externally by others. As control is transferred from teacher to child, higher-order executive processes become internalized and self-perception improves. Given that transcription skills play a key role in written expression, it is useful to provide alternative strategies such as computer literacy to assist developing writers with the executive functions necessary for proficient writing skills.

Steven G. Feifer, Ed.S., NCSP    Philip A. De Fina, Ph.D., ABPdN

# The 90 minute Dysgraphia Evaluation

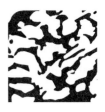

# Chapter 8

"Imagination is more important than knowledge."
— Albert Einstein

The human genome project has identified some 3 billion base pairs of DNA, comprising approximately 30,000 genes that transcribe the chemical messages from which a human being is made. Amazingly, there are only 200,000 base pairs of DNA that differentiate one individual from the next. Still, relatively subtle chemical differences in genotype produce immense differences in the observable expression of behavior (phenotype). For instance, human beings are genetically 99.6 % similar to chimpanzees, a figure that makes us more similar to a simian population than rats are to mice (Sagan, 1980). Many of these differences involve the neuronal distribution of the cerebral cortex and the development of the prefrontal lobes, which of course is the seat for higher-level cognitive skills. According to Steven Hyman, director of the National Institute of Mental Health,

*"For every complex behavioral trait investigated, from learning disabilities to risk of mental illness, multiple genes each of which contribute a small increment of influence coupled with non-genetic environmental factors interact to produce a trait. Science is very much*

*interested in discovering genes related to behavior that create risks of learning and/or mental illness."*

Numerous disciplines ranging from molecular biology to cognitive neuroscience must carry out the daunting task of evaluating subtle differences in brain functioning. Today, the recipients of such powerful information are in most part educators, who daily face the unenviable challenge of changing brain chemistry through systematic instruction in order to produce academic growth, a process known as education. Of course, the real payoff of the human genome project is identifying genes implicated in psychiatric and physical disorders so that treatments can be geared toward altering biochemical networks before these maladaptive behavioral traits emerge. Similarly, psychologists and educators need a methodology to identify students at risk for reading and written language disorders systematically so that interventions may take place before more permanent learning dysfunction occurs. In other words, the current *wait and fail* policy that drives educational placement decisions needs to be replaced by a more proactive methodology that identifies students as being at-risk much earlier in their academic careers. Unfortunately, recent data reported in 2001 by the National Institute of Child Health and Human Development (NICHD) indicated that 20% of elementary school students are at risk for reading and written language failure. Furthermore, 74% of students identified as having a learning disability by the third grade continue to require special education services through the ninth grade as well (Lyon, 1996). One reason for this abysmal statistic is that students need to be identified much earlier than the third grade, when interventions are much more likely to be effective and the brain is more receptive to linguistically based interventions. Notwithstanding these statistics, no student should have to forego years of academic futility and failure before qualifying for assistance.

According to statistics compiled by the Maryland State Department of Education from the 2000-2001 school year, 628 school psychologists conducted over 52,000 assessments, with the average psychologist performing some 83 evaluations per year spread among four schools. With demand for psychological and educational assessments reaching epic proportions, psychologists tend to complete most evaluations in just a single testing session with minimal assessment instruments used. Assembly line testing has become the norm, meaning that educational institutions make critical decisions regarding the life and education of a child more hastily and with less information. A *fixed battery* approach is often the norm in school-based assessments, meaning that a pre-selected battery of instruments is used to conduct an evaluation regardless of the referral question. Thus, students suspected of a learning disability or autism, of mental retardation or emotional disturbance, of speech and language impairments or clinical depression, all receive similar diagnostic work-ups. It's as though the rainbow of colors that comprise the emotional and cognitive spectrum is viewed through a single black and white lens. Very rarely are test batteries tailored or adjusted in a substantial manner to answer the specifics of the referral question.

There are three primary reasons for such a mechanistic approach towards psycho-educational assessment. First, a lack of sufficient time drives many psychological assessments, with most examiners relying on instruments with which they are most comfortable in order to speed up their productivity. Second, most assessments tend to be *administrative assessments* and not clinical in nature. In this capacity, evaluations only need to meet the local criterion for justifying a handicapping condition, thus allowing access to special education services. Consequently, there is no need to delve into a more tertiary analysis of why a given behavior occurs. This leads to test batteries that reflect bureaucratic educational policies and criteria, as opposed to clinically based assessments depicting the interplay of memory, attention, language, visual-spatial skills, and temperament in contributing toward success or failure on a given cognitive task. Third, many psychologists simply lack sufficient training in brain-behavioral analysis to describe mental functions and cognitive events in those terms.

As psychologists and educators head into the 21st century, a new paradigm for assessing children seems of vital importance in order to assist educators in remediating learning disorders in children. Ideally, such an approach should be:

- flexible enough to adapt to the behavioral or cognitive issues in question;
- capable of identifying students at earlier ages;
- performed in a timely manner; and
- based upon brain-behavioral relationships which lead to meaningful interventions.

As mentioned previously, the scope and stature of a psycho-educational assessment often is centered on addressing the issue of eligibility for special education services as opposed to linking the specific neurodevelopmental strengths and weaknesses of a child with effective interventions. One of the great paradoxes in special education remains the notion of an Individualized Education Plan (IEP), as most goals and objectives are merely frequently recycled templates and not plans tailored to or individualized for the needs of the child. Furthermore, the illusion remains that simply writing down on paper the desired goal or expectation for student achievement, without detailing how to accomplish the goal, somehow constitutes an intervention. For instance, stating that Johnny will write a complete sentence with 75% of the words spelled correctly on eight out of 10 occasions is a worthy goal. However, without some instruction as to how to accomplish this goal, the IEP almost mocks the regular education teacher who no doubt already had similar expectations for Johnny but who does not know how to achieve this objective.

To accomplish the ambitious endeavor of evaluating students from a brain-behavioral perspective, a *flexible battery* or *cross battery* approach that tests specific psychological constructs is needed. In other words, rather than administering one test from start to finish such as the *NEPSY* (which takes approximately 90 minutes), specific subtests should be administered which would measure the specific psychological construct in question most effectively. For instance, if the referral question involves language processing issues, perhaps only three subtests from the *NEPSY (phonological awareness tests, rapid naming tests, and comprehension of instructions)*, each of which takes 3-5 minutes to administer, should be given rather than the entire 14-subtest battery. The ability to pick and choose various subtests from a variety of instruments not only tailors an evaluation to the individual needs of the child but also maximizes the ability of psychologists to test various cognitive domains in a brief span of time. Nevertheless, the true advantage of a flexible battery approach is the power and precision with which information can be analyzed in order to determine the integrity of specific neural pathways necessary to perform a given cognitive task. Therefore, psychologists need to evaluate the data from multiple methods of inferences as opposed to just a *level of performance* approach. According to Jarvis and Barth (1994), the following taxonomy represents how a school-based neuropsychologist can best analyze test results from a brain-behavioral perspective:

# TABLE 8-1

## Four methods of inference to analyze Data

1. **Level of Performance** – total score on a given measure. For instance, evaluating intelligence on the basis of a single IQ score. Often a generalized measure, yielding limited data on individual strengths and weaknesses.

2. **Patterns of Performance** – evaluating how a score was determined by examining the relationship between scores and a given construct. Thus, if a student's Verbal IQ was somewhat low, and scores on reading and written language were consistently low as well, then solid evidence increases the probability of a language processing deficit.

3. **Functioning of Two Sides of Body** – many psychological functions are distributed in both left and right hemisphere responsibilities as well as by anterior and posterior responsibilities.

4. **Pathognomonic Signs** – extreme deficits such as an unusually low test score; writing that is abnormally large, small, or bunched to one side of the page; or deficits in copying are suggestive of neurological impairment.

*Adapted from Jarvis, P.E., & Barth, J.T., (1994). *The Halstead-Reitan neuropsychological test battery: A guide to interpretation and clinical applications*. Odessa, FL: Psychological Assessment Resources.

The ultimate goal of any evaluation goes beyond providing an exposition of a student's unique learning profile. Rather, it must serve as a bridge to effective remediation techniques. By adopting a neuropsychological paradigm, psychologists can truly individualize interventions based on the developing neural pathways that modulate a given cognitive task. As the neuroscientific community slowly unravels the mysteries behind human cognitive functioning, educators now find themselves in a position to synchronize curriculum expectations with the developing brain of a child. The timing of specific teaching practices during critical *learning windows* in brain development should yield more efficacious outcomes for special education programs. In summary, Table 8-2 provides an overview of a flexible battery approach for assessing students with written language difficulties in a single testing session - namely, the 90 minute dysgraphia evaluation.

## TABLE 8-2

### The 90 Minute Dysgraphia Evaluation

1. **INTELLIGENCE MEASURES:**
   - Wechsler Intelligence Scales for Children
   - Cognitive Assessment System
   - Differential Ability Scales
   - Woodcock-Johnson III

2. **CONSTRUCTIONAL DYSPRAXIA:**
   - Beery Visual-Motor Integration Test
   - Bender Gestalt
   - NEPSY (Design Copying)
   - Process Assessment of the Learner (Copying)
   - Wide Range Assessment of Visual Motor Abilities
   - Rey Complex Figure Test

3. **WORKING MEMORY:**
   - Test of Memory and Learning (Digits and Letters Backwards)
   - Trailmaking Test (Halstead-Reitan)
   - Planned Connections (Cognitive Assessment System)
   - Children's Memory Scale (Dot Locations and Sequences)
   - Woodcock Johnson III (Auditory Working Memory)
   - WISC PI ( Spatial span, Arithmetic & Sentence Arrangement)
   - Wechsler Memory Scale (Visual reproduction & Paired Associate)
   - Paced Auditory Serial Addition Test (PASAT)
   - Wide Range Assessment of Memory and Learning (Finger Windows)

4. **EXECUTIVE FUNCTIONS:**
   - Wisconsin Card Sort Test
   - Stroop Test
   - BRIEF (Behavior Rating Inventory of Executive Functions)
   - Brown ADD Scales for Children (3-12)
   - Woodcock Johnson III (Planning)
   - Cognitive Assessment System (Planned Connections)
   - Delis-Kaplan Executive Function Scale
   - NEPSY (Tower)
   - WISC PI (Elithorn Mazes)
   - Booklet Category Test for Children

5. **WRITING AND SPELLING SKILLS:**
   - Wechsler Individual Achievement Test- 2nd Edition
   - Woodcock Johnson III
   - Test of Written Language-3rd Edition (TOWL-3)
   - Test of Written Spelling-4th Edition

| Steven G. Feifer, Ed.S., NCSP    Philip A. De Fina, Ph.D., ABPdN

- Test of Early Written Language –2nd Edition (TEWL-2)
- Test of Written Expression (TOWE)
- OWLS Written Expression Scale
- Informal Writing Assessment

## 6. PHONOLOGICAL AWARENESS TESTS:

- Comprehensive Test of Phonological Processing (C-TOPP)
- Process Assessment of the Learner (Phonemes & Pseudo-word Decoding)
- Woodcock-Johnson III (Word Attack)
- Phonological Awareness Test
- NEPSY (Phonological Processing)
- Test of Word Reading Efficiency (TOWRE)

## 7. RETRIEVAL FLUENCY MEASURES:

- Woodcock-Johnson III (Retrieval Fluency & Rapid Picture Naming)
- NEPSY (Verbal Fluency & Speeded Coding)
- Process Assessment of the Learner (Expressive Coding & Sentence Sense)
- Controlled Oral Word Association Test (COWAT)

## 8. FAMILY HISTORY:

*Intelligence Tests:* A ubiquitous definition of *intelligence* per se remains somewhat elusive, as do the nature of "g" and the precision with which higher level thinking and problem solving skills can truly be quantified. Nevertheless, intelligence tests remain the single best predictor for success in school and play a pivotal role in the clinical assessment of a child. However, rather than interpreting intelligence measures from a singular method of inference - namely, overall performance - specific patterns of performance should be analyzed to further assess the nature of a particular deficit.

Since two-thirds of all students will score within one standard deviation of the mean (85 -115), the skilled examiner must go further in dissecting subtle processing cues to determine specific breakdowns in the written language process. For instance, with respect to the *WISC-III*, the cluster of subtests that comprise the *Verbal IQ* score can be compared with the cluster of subtests that comprise the Performance *IQ* scores to determine whether or not deficits in written language stem from more linguistic based reasons or from poor motor output. Once again, discrepancies between verbal and performance skills of up to 15 points are perfectly normal within the cognitive landscape of a child and not automatically reflective of a disability (Kaufman, 1994). Therefore, simply relying upon an *overall* score yields limited information about specific problem solving skills, and has reduced clinical value unless a student scores at the extreme end of the distribution. From an item analysis standpoint, Table 8-3 summarizes various interpretation strategies when examining the relationship between individual subtest scores and their potential relationship toward deficits in the writing process.

## TABLE 8-3

| cognitive subtest Measures and written Language | | |
|---|---|---|
| Intelligence Measure | subtest | sub-skill of written Language |
| WISC III | Information | Word retrieval skills |
| WISC III | Similarities | Conceptual word knowledge and usage |
| WISC III | Arithmetic | Active working memory |
| WISC III | Vocabulary | General lexicon of words |
| WISC III | Comprehension | Verbal syntax skills and divergent thinking skills. |
| WISC III | Digits Forward | Auditory attention and short-term memory |
| WISC III | Digits Backwards | Active working memory |
| WISC III | Picture Completion | Nonverbal responses suggest limited word finding skills |
| WISC III | Coding | Visual-motor speed and visual sketchpad component of active working memory |
| WISC III | Picture Arrangement | Sequencing and planning skills along with executive functioning |
| WISC III | Block Design | Breakdown in details reflects poor attention to visual detail |
| | | Breakdown in pattern of matrix suggest poor executive functioning |
| CAS | Expressive Attention | Similar to stroop test in measuring executive functioning and ability to ignore competing responses |
| CAS | Planned Codes | Visual-motor speed and visual sketchpad component of active working memory |
| CAS | Planned Connections | Active working memory skills |
| CAS | Figure Memory | Measures visual-spatial and praxic skill |
| CAS | Word Series | Short-term memory skills |
| CAS | Sentence Repetition | Short-term memory skills |
| WJIII | Verbal Comprehension | Lexical knowledge |
| WJIII | Visual-Auditory Learning | Word retrieval skills |

| WJIII | Spatial Relations | Visual-spatial reasoning skills |
|---|---|---|
| WJIII | Concept Formation | Fluid reasoning, executive functioning skills |
| WJIII | Visual Matching | Visual-motor speed |
| WJIII | Sound Blending | Phonological awareness |
| WJIII | Numbers Reversed | Working memory |
| WJIII | Incomplete Words | Phonological awareness |
| WJIII | Auditory Working Memory | Working memory |

***Constructional Dyspraxia:*** The evaluation of any written language endeavor ultimately depends on the analysis of some output or production by a student. This can be accomplished through both formal and informal means. The first notation by any qualified diagnostician should involve the handedness of the child, with the second notation being a brief description of pencil grip. The Schneck and Henderson (1990) grip scale, depicted in Table 5-1, provides an excellent guideline for determining the efficacy of pencil grip.

However, the importance of handedness cannot be emphasized enough. Nearly 90 percent of the population is right-handed, and therefore most of their linguistic skills are housed within the architecture of the left hemisphere. For left-handers, nearly two-thirds have linguistic representation in the left hemisphere, while the remaining one-third have either bilateral representation of language skills or right-hemispheric dominance for language. Since special education has encountered an overabundance of left-handers identified with a learning disability, perhaps left-handedness reflects some subtle abnormality in the development of the left hemisphere, thereby resulting in right hemispheric dominance for both motor skills and linguistic functioning. As mentioned previously, there are numerous limitations with the right hemisphere's linguistic prowess, most visibly indicated by poor syntax skills and limited phonological awareness (Ogden, 1996). As a final note, *pathological left-handedness* refers to children who are left-handed when both parents are strongly right-handed. This occurs just 2 percent of the time, indicating that these children may have been biologically destined to become right-handed but became left-handed due to deficits in the developing left hemisphere. In any event, forming a conceptual hypothesis for how information is stored, processed, accessed, and organized is the first step for any neuropsychologist.

A third observation worth noting involves the actual layout of the handwritten page coupled with the quality of the printed information. Certainly, both micrographia (excessively small writing) and macrographia (extremely large writing) have neurological implications. Additionally, writing that is bunched to the right side of the page may reflect neglect, a phenomena of right parietal lobe damage. The tidiness of print can be affected by numerous factors including fatigue, anxiety, emotional issues, motivation, and, of course, fine motor coordination. Multiple writing samples should be ascertained during different times of the day to develop a baseline writing sample. Table 8-2 lists specific objective measures that can be used in part to determine the presence of a motor skill dyspraxia.

***Working Memory:***   The performance of any routine task, such as talking with a neighbor or following directions from a recipe, requires some element of working memory skills. In school, the ability to juggle multiple cognitive demands at once - listening and taking notes, reading and comprehending, writing sentences to convey our thoughts - comes under the direct command of our working memory systems. However, this critically important component of written language is among the constructs most frequently overlooked by psychologists when evaluating learning deficits in children. Working memory, which relies heavily upon the skilled precision of the prefrontal cortex, provides a uniquely human quality - namely, the ability to multi-task. Working memory allows students to recall spelling rules, sentence structures, punctuation variations, and syntax simultaneously in order to organize their thoughts on paper. When teachers lament that some students can spell words perfectly in isolation but struggle when spelling the same word within the context of a paragraph, the culprit is often working memory. In essence, there is a mismatch between the cognitive workspace needed to recall multiple memory processes (e.g., spelling, syntax, grammar, etc.) required by the demands of the task and the working memory available. Unfortunately, anxiety remains a leading culprit in reducing the size of working memory even further, leading to a vicious cycle for students with fears about essay tests. Often, these students have difficulty initiating a written response as anxiety shrinks their cognitive workspace, thus limiting their ability to dedicate enough attention resources to the multi-level task of written expression. There are three subcomponents comprising our working memory store that need to be addressed during the evaluation process.

First, the memory span for ***phonological information,*** which tends to be stored in a sequential manner, should be evaluated. According to Baddeley (2000), the following factors should be taken into consideration when evaluating the phonological memory span:

1. ***Similarity Effect*** – Items such as letters that are similar in sound are harder to remember. Thus, sequencing the letters *g,c,b,r,v,p* is harder than remembering dissimilar letter sounds such as *f,w,k,s,y.*

2. ***Word-Length Effect*** – Students find it easier to recall a sequence of short words *(fun, hit, bag, top)* than longer words *(graduation, opportunity, ideology).* Since it takes longer to rehearse the polysyllables in the longer words, they are more prone to decay.

3. ***Articulatory Suppression*** – Students prevented from rehearsing items to be remembered show declining performances. Words not subvocalized or rehearsed are quickly forgotten.

4. ***Attentional Strength*** – Mental fatigue, distractibility, and anxiety are significant detractors of attention resources that hinder the memory store.

Second, the ***visual-spatial sketchpad*** is a secondary sub-system of working memory that allows visual and spatial characteristics to be temporarily preserved for future recall. For instance, in recalling the correct spelling of a word, proper tense structures, and punctuation rules as well as grammatical aspects of sentences, students often rely in part on visual cues to assist with recall. In other words, drawing a mental image of how a word is spelled or how a sentence should look comes under the purview of the visual-spatial sketchpad. In addition, students who have difficulty judging how large their handwriting should be in order to fit the parameters of the page, misjudge margins, have unusual spacing between words and letters, and demonstrate poor use of lines may have difficulty with this element of working memory. Lastly, ***surface dysgraphia***, which is characterized by poor knowledge of the idiosyncratic properties of words, e.g., poor lexical representations (Romani, et. al., 1999), may be strongly associated with a faulty visual-spatial sketchpad.

In summary, when assessing working memory, psychologists should choose specific measures that tap both ***phonological*** and ***visual-spatial*** processes, in addition to noting a student's preferred mode of memory storage. For instance, students who tend to subvocalize and rehearse out loud while attempting to write are probably over-relying on their phonological processes. On the other hand, students who write down items on a page only to erase their efforts and reconstruct their thoughts yet again may have difficulty maintaining information in their visual-spatial sketchpad. In this case, written information must first be created on paper for the mind to see before it can be modified, edited, and reworked to fit the parameters of the assignment.

Lastly, the **central executive system** oversees the interaction between both the phonological and visual-spatial working memory systems and plays an important role in determining which strategy a student uses while problem solving. The ability to oversee two or more tasks remains an essential feature of the central executive system and often is dependent upon frontal lobe functioning (Baddeley, 1998). Therefore, practitioners should be cautious in their assessment when differentiating skills completed in isolation versus those within the context of written expression. For instance, the **Woodcock-Johnson III** requires a student to spell a word in isolation, or punctuate a word in isolation, or determine a specific tense or grammatical feature of a word in isolation. While some students may have little difficulty executing these tasks in isolation, e.g., in an individual test-taking situation, they may struggle with accurately completing their written work on a daily basis within the context of a classroom. In all likelihood, the deficit lies in the inability of the central executive component to allocate enough attention resources to each individual subcomponent of the writing process.

***Executive Functioning:*** The ability to self-monitor written work may be the most critical feature of accomplished writing, especially for older students. The passage must be constantly monitored to determine if the piece is suitable for the intended audience, whether the tone and language are appropriate, and whether it conforms to the structural requirements of the composition. The ability to review their written work allows students to monitor their own effectiveness as communicators and evaluate their own skill level in meeting the goals of an assignment. As noted previously, students with an attention-deficit-disorder often struggle with many aspects of the written language process, as their impulsive cognitive style precludes them from self-monitoring their written production. Therefore, a prudent examiner may want to determine if there is a co-existing attentional deficit when work production is sloppy, careless, and filled with numerous errors. Since formal testing of executive functioning can be rather elusive, the following behaviors noted in Table 7-1 should be assessed informally through observation of work samples or by teacher interviews to tease out the salient features of this domain. If a suspected deficit is present, formal testing such as those instruments listed in Table 8-2 may be helpful in explaining and remediating written language deficits.

***Writing and Spelling Skills:*** Table 8-2 lists a variety of formalized tests that rely on a national normative sample to determine both the age and grade level of a student's written language prowess. However, the skilled examiner may find that a qualitative analysis of written language and spelling skills may yield more promising results than a quantitative one. For instance, an error analysis of misspelled words can assist in determining the specific subtype of dysgraphia. The hallmark feature of ***phonological dysgraphia*** is an over-reliance on the visual features of words and inability to spell pseudowords. On the other hand, the primary characteristic of ***surface dysgraphia*** is an over-reliance on the sound patterns of words, reflecting a relatively poor understanding of the idiosyncratic properties of the English language. In other words, some students rely on the individual sound patterns of words when spelling, while others utilize their own mental dictionary to conjure up what a given word looks like in the mind's eye.

Perhaps the greatest advantage of evaluating individual writing skills from a qualitative perspective is the ability to link specific test outcomes with effective remediation techniques. Simply regurgitating a singular intelligence test score or the standard score on a particular writing measure may assist educators in determining in which category of special education a student may fit. However, it yields virtually meaningless data for the development of an effective Individualized Education Plan (IEP). Consequently, IEP's in the school system tend to become rather generic and somewhat indistinguishable, with most goals and objectives being similar for all students despite marked differences in the neurodevelopmental profile of the learner. While there are numerous reasons for failure of special education to remediate deficient academic skills effectively, poor IEP development stemming from incomplete psycho-educational evaluations remains a significant factor. Therefore, a thorough evaluation of the writing and spelling process should include increased emphasis on syntax, grammar, elaboration, word usage, fluency, and organization, as opposed to overall test scores. This should yield far more information that educators can utilize to determine both the subtype of dysgraphia and the selection of specific remediation techniques. In addition, observing the placement of words on the paper, the spacing of words and letters, and handwriting fluency and grip will also assist in determining the presence of a non-language type of dysgraphia as well.

Finally, the mode of presentation – e.g., oral spelling versus copying, spontaneous writing versus structured writing, and writing to dictation versus free-form writing - should be noted in the evaluative process. Often, students with poor working memory skills have difficulty taking notes in a lecture-oriented class setting, although they may perform better on more prosaic types of writing tasks. Additionally, some students with executive functioning difficulties may have difficulty writing on command and struggle on most classroom writing activities, but perform better when inspired or motivated when writing for pleasure. A thorough evaluation of writing and spelling skills should evaluate the writing process not just from a motor output perspective, but should also examine the mode of presentation to determine exactly where the breakdown lies with respect to written production.

***Phonological Awareness Skills:*** There is considerable evidence that a primary cause of variability among children acquiring early literacy skills involves individual differences in the ability to process the phonological features of language (Torgesen & Hecht, 1996). In the school-age child, the most important element of the psychometric evaluation of dyslexia is how accurately a child can decode words (Shaywitz, 1998). Countless studies have shown that the single best predictor of reading difficulty in kindergarten and first grade is phonological awareness, not intelligence test scores (Hurford, et. al, 1994, Lyon, 1996). Knowledge of the alphabetic code allows children to use linguistic and auditory cues independently to break down unfamiliar words. Two distinct forms of phonological processing apparently exist that need to be teased out in the evaluation process. The first involves just rote level phonics - pairing an isolated sound with a symbol. From a neuropsychological perspective, the functional integrity of the ***plana temporale*** in the left hemisphere is key to successful classification of sound patterns with symbols. The second type is a higher-level phonemic awareness skill that includes a metacognitive understanding of word boundaries, syllable boundaries, and the isolation and segmentation of phonemes within a given word (Clark & Uhry, 1995). Some of these tests might involve rhyming activities, sound blending, sound segmenting, and reading and decoding nonwords. The seat of visual-verbal learning and higher-level manipulation of phonemes in print lies mainly in the ***angular gyrus*** of the left hemisphere, a posterior brain region where the occipital and temporal lobes interface.

According to Moats (1993), 90 percent of a high school student's spelling errors can be attributed to faulty phonological awareness skills. Phonological errors have traditionally been defined by adding, omitting, shifting, or repeating phonemes in words during reading or when spelling. Even in kindergarten, valuable predictors for later literacy deficits include problems in phonological awareness, language comprehension skills, and mastery of letter names with their corresponding sounds. The ability to master the corresponding sound patterns that comprise some 30,000 common words in the average English lexicon lies at the heart of future reading and writing success. In essence, good writers must be able to apply language patterns that are similar to those used by good readers - namely, comparable letter shapes, sentence structure, syntax, and sound-symbol associations. Based upon research by Bailet (2001), Table 8-4 details the typical developmental sequence in which children acquire phonological awareness skills:

## TABLE 8-4

| developmental progression of phonemic awareness skills | |
|---|---|
| AGE | SKILL MASTERY |
| 3 | Reciting nursery rhymes |
| 4 | Detecting and categorizing rhyming words |
| 5 | Count syllables and phonemes in words |
| 6 | Basic sound-symbol association and inventive spelling |
| 7 | Sound blending and manipulation of phonemes (i.e. Substitute "g" for "t" in the word "*tame*" and what is left?) |
| 8 | Sound categorization through print and ability to spell nonwords |
| 9-12 | Rapid and automatic recognition of sound patterns. |

***Retrieval Fluency Skills:*** Perhaps more than any other cognitive skill, written language requires the harmonious synchronization of multiple perceptual and lexical processes, thus placing undue importance on the ability to retrieve information effectively into active working memory. According to Levine (1999), children with written language deficits tend to show erratic patterns of retrieval memory and fluency, and may be prone to uneven recall of the motor engrams necessary to form letters and words. In fact, observing a child write from dictation may serve as an excellent means of noting hesitations stemming from the rapid recall of vocabulary, syntax, spelling rules, and grammar. The fluency and speed of a student's access to linguistic information from memory stores play a vital role in the development and mastery of literacy skills. According to a five-year longitudinal study by Maryanne Wolf (1999), a preeminent researcher in the field of dyslexia, naming speed for children with reading disabilities was visible from the first day of kindergarten. In fact, retrieval speed and fluency were found to be a better predictor of literacy deficits than poor phonological awareness skills. This was especially evident in more orthographically consistent languages such as German, Dutch, Finnish, and Spanish. As Wolf (1999) noted:

*Naming speed deficits accompany dyslexia and dysgraphia in many children in many language systems because naming speed is a mini, multi-componential version of reading. Retrieval fluency represents ensembles of multiple perceptual, lexical, and motoric processes, all the subprocesses of which must function smoothly and rapidly in order to produce a verbal match for an abstract, visually oriented symbol. (Wolf, p.12)*

Unlike reading, the written language process requires access to words without the luxury of an external visual cue. Writers of all skill levels are plagued by the never-ending challenge of selecting a precise word among thousands of possible candidates to convey their internal thought process effectively. There are no tour guides or external access cues to navigate the hierarchical fashion by which the brain categorizes language. Written language requires the rapid and automatic retrieval of language based simply upon the cumulative recall of prior learning experiences. For instance, if asked to make an entry into a diary, the skilled writer must mentally go back in time to allow the proper sequence of events from a given day to unfold in an unfettered fashion. Thus, multiple memory processes are activated to allow the writer to recall this information in a particular order. If linguistic retrieval skills are not fully automatized, more cognitive energy must be devoted to this process, reducing the efficiency of other memory processes as well. The net result is a poorly detailed account of the day's events, chalked by an awkward flow of ideas.

While most students rely heavily on internal semantic cues to retrieve specific lexical information, the skilled writer often uses phonological cues as well. For instance, when attempting to think of a word meaning *"knowledge"*, most students tend to come up with words such as *"data"*," *facts*", *"information"*," *intelligence*", or *"wisdom"*. However, words such as *"know-how"* or *"know-it-all"* may also arise for those using the prefix *"know"* to scan for other similar sounding words with consistent meanings. Consequently, using a variety of strategies to bring multiple words into working memory adds fluency and precision to the written language process. Therefore, the prudent examiner should tease out the strategy employed by the student to retrieve specific words from memory. One effective measure that assists in discriminating word retrieval strategy is the *Verbal Fluency* subtest from the *NEPSY*. Students are asked to name as many animals or types of foods as possible in a minute. Next, students must come up with as many words beginning with the letters *"f"* or *"s"* in a minute. Many students with dysgraphia have extreme difficulty using phonological cues (letters) to retrieve words from memory and seem to over-rely on semantic categories (i.e. animals or foods) for word recall. Educators may find that teaching mnemonic strategies, which assist students in using visual imagery to both store and retrieve information, may aid with word retrieval skills by providing yet another access route to our memory stores for language.

From a neuropsychological perspective, multiple brain regions are responsible for the ability to retrieve specific words instantly from our cognitive archives to convey our thoughts in print. After all, the brain has 100 trillion connections joining billions of neurons with each junction having the potential to be part of the human memory store (Carter, 1998). Still, there appears to be functional hemispheric specialization for specific forms of memory (Jodzio, 1995). Specifically, the left hemisphere plays a vital role in the retrieval process of language, though subcortical areas such as the limbic system with its rich interconnections with both the temporal lobes and prefrontal cortex have been implicated as well (Jodzio, 1995). The **hippocampus** is intricately linked to both the storage and retrieval of factual-based memories and plays an important role in the conscious recall of a specific word. Under conditions of stress or anxiety, such as an important test or when called upon to respond to a question in front of the entire class, stress hormones may be released in such abundance that hippocampal functioning becomes impaired and retrieval skills are compromised. Therefore, most writers who seek inspirational settings to practice their craft are really searching for a tranquil and stress-free environment to maximize the fluidity by which their brains can retrieve linguistic concepts. In the classroom, most students will perform better under more calm and placid conditions where stress is kept to a minimal.

**Family History:** There is a paucity of data regarding the degree with which dysgraphia runs in families. Still, most clinicians have long been convinced that dyslexia runs in families. Most genetic studies examining dyslexia suggest that both normal reading and written language ability are significantly influenced by heredity, though the precise mode of genetic transmission may vary tremendously. According to Pennington (1995), approximately 27% to 49% of parents and 40% of siblings of children are affected to some degree. In fact, a child with an affected parent has an approximately **eightfold** increase in risk compared with the approximate 5 % risk found in the normal population.

Research carried out as part of the Colorado twin study indicated that in 70% of cases involving identical twins, when one twin had a learning disability, the other did as well. However, in cases involving fraternal twins the concordance rate was only about 48% (DeFries et al., 1991). Interestingly, this study suggested a strong genetic influence among phonological skills, though this was not the case with orthographic skills. These researchers concluded that learning disabilities were both *familial*, with approximately 40% of first-degree relatives affected, and *heritable*, with a transmission rate of approximately 50%. Further studies have focused on a possible dyslexic gene, with chromosome 6 and chromosome 15 being possible candidates. However, this research is still in its infancy, and to date, no specific gene for dyslexia or dysgraphia has been found. In any event, there appears to be a genetic factor for both dyslexia and dysgraphia, and as with virtually any psychological evaluation, a detailed developmental history with maximum parental input remains essential.

# case study: Jeremy

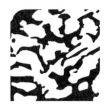

# Chapter 9

"genius not only diagnosis the situation but also supplies the answers."
— oscar wilde

**REASON FOR REFERRAL:** Jeremy was referred for a neuropsychological evaluation due to continued difficulty acquiring basic reading and written language skills, in addition to a persistent pattern of intractable learning problems. Assessment was administered in order to determine his future educational needs.

**BACKGROUND INFORMATION:** Jeremy is a 10-year-old student currently in the 5th grade at Hunt Valley Elementary School. He was referred for a complete evaluation due to continued difficulty acquiring basic reading and written language skills in addition to a persistent pattern of intractable learning problems. A brief review of his academic records indicated that Jeremy was initially evaluated for special education services in October 1998 while in 2nd grade at Hunt Valley Elementary School. At the time, there were concerns regarding his inability to master the alphabet, recognize letters in his name, and learn basic sound-symbol correspondences. There were additional concerns regarding his attention and concentration in class. It should be noted that Jeremy had been diagnosed as having Attention-Deficit-Disorder the previous year, though he had discontinued his medication.

The test results indicated his overall cognitive skills were in the Low Average range of functioning (FSIQ=88), with significant weaknesses noted with phonemic awareness skills as well as short-term memory skills. Further testing revealed that he failed to identify words on a page accurately, struggled with basic letter identification skills, and often used external cues (finger counting) or subvocalizations (verbal rehearsal) when solving math problems. Jeremy was found eligible for special education services as a learning disabled student. He also qualified for speech and language services due to poor syntactical awareness skills. There were no behavioral issues reported, as Jeremy was described as being a pleasant and cooperative student who interacted well with both peers and adults.

Since his initial evaluation, the school reported that Jeremy had made virtually no educational progress while in special education, despite numerous remediation strategies and modifications attempted by the school. These included:

- Phonemic awareness training
- Alphabetic Phonics instruction
- Lindamood Program: Auditory Discrimination in Depth
- Lindamood Program: Sounds abound
- Repetitive tests and pattern books at instructional level
- Developmental spelling program
- Varied language experiences
- Small group instruction
- Adaptations to tests and assignments (dictation, tests read to him, etc.)

In spite of these interventions, Jeremy still could not recognize all of the letters in the alphabet, and continued to read on an approximately pre-primer level. His overall written language skills were extremely limited as well. Additional concerns regarded his limited memory skills, wandering attention span, and poor word finding skills.

**DEVELOPMENTAL HISTORY:** A brief review of Jeremy's developmental history indicated he currently resides with both parents and one younger brother who also receives special education services. According to his mother, Jeremy was born full term, with no reported birth complications or difficulties with pregnancy noted. Still, Jeremy was described as being somewhat late in reaching most developmental milestones with respect to walking, talking, and toileting skills. His mother mentioned that Jeremy also contracted numerous ear infections during toddlerhood. He was frequently given antibiotics, and eventually had tubes placed in his ears. There were no reports of prolonged high fevers, head injuries, accidents, or seizure activity. Jeremy's father was reported as having significant learning disabilities with respect to reading and written language, and also received special education services.

Jeremy's parents have expressed significant concerns regarding his lack of educational progress, and are somewhat frustrated by his unusual learning habits. For instance, his mother indicated Jeremy was able to spell aloud much better than on paper, and often failed most spelling tests despite knowing the words when quizzed at home. In addition, handedness had always been an issue, as he initially appeared to be right-handed, though he tended to switch handedness periodically. According to his father, Jeremy appeared to be cross-dominant as he preferred to hunt left-handed, though used his dominant right eye to align the target. Furthermore, he tended to bat either right-handed or left-handed when playing baseball. The school eventually forced him to choose a preferred hand when writing, and he chose his left hand. Despite his learning limitations, Jeremy was described as enjoying school, and particularly enjoyed working with computers. His overall math skills were described as being an area of strength, though he continued to write numbers backwards.

**BEHAVIOR OBSERVATIONS:** Jeremy appeared to be of medium stature for his age with short brown hair and an earring. He was extremely upbeat and cheerful in his manner, and seemed to thrive on the one-on-one attention he was receiving. Jeremy warmed up quickly to the assessment process, and rapport was easily established and maintained. His overall response style to most questions was normally paced and not hurried or rushed. Jeremy demonstrated a very positive learning temperament, putting forth an outstanding effort, readily attempting most problem solving tasks, and not becoming frustrated or discouraged by more challenging items. His overall speech and language skills seemed age-appropriate, with no specific word finding deficits, syntactical confusion, or dysphasias evident at this time.

Jeremy was extremely candid and forthright in his manner, and readily acknowledged his academic deficiencies. He cordially attempted to read and write independently when asked to do so, despite marked limitations in these areas. Jeremy exhibited a strong left-handed dominance throughout the evaluation, and tended to hold his pencil perfectly straight, as if he were gripping and throwing a dart. In fact, he asked to use a pencil, and mentioned he had difficulty controlling and manipulating a pen. Jeremy had little difficulty focusing his attention or sustaining his concentration in a one-on-one setting. There were no signs of hyperactivity or excess motor activity hindering his skills or abilities. In sum, Jeremy appeared to put forth his best during this evaluation, and the following results should be a valid and reliable estimate of his skills and abilities.

*INTELLIGENCE TEST MEASURES:* Jeremy was given the **WISC-III** in order to assess his overall level of cognitive functioning. This test measures two unique styles of information processing and problem solving. The **Verbal IQ** subtests assess a student's verbal ability, general knowledge base, and language development skills. The **Performance IQ** subtests assess nonverbal reasoning and visual perceptual skills as well as speed of information processing. Both the verbal and performance subtests combine to yield an overall or Full Scale score. *The reader should be cautioned that intelligence tests do not measure important attributes for learning such as creativity, motivation to learn, or personality styles, though they remain an excellent predictor of academic success.*

Jeremy's **Full Scale IQ** was in the lower end of the *Average* range of functioning, at the **27**th percentile compared to peers. His **Verbal IQ** was in the *Low Average* range, at the **16**th percentile, while his **Performance IQ** was in the *Average* range, at the **47**th percentile compared to peers. *The difference between his verbal and nonverbal problem solving skills was not significant.* The rest of his domain scores were as follows:

| verbal | ss | performance | ss |
|---|---|---|---|
| Information | 6 | Picture Completion | 11 |
| Similarities | 9 | Coding | 6 |
| Arithmetic | 4 | Picture Arrangement | 9 |
| Vocabulary | 9 | Block Design | 12 |
| Comprehension | 9 | Object Assembly | 11 |
| Digit Span | 3 | Symbol Search | 9 |
| | | | (Mean = 10) |

| | | RANGE |
|---|---|---|
| Verbal IQ: | 85 ( 80 - 92) | LOW AVERAGE |
| Performance IQ: | 99 ( 91 - 107) | AVERAGE |
| Full Scale IQ: | 91 ( 86 – 97) | AVERAGE |

Within the verbal domain, Jeremy demonstrated adequate language development and verbal comprehension skills. He had little difficulty defining individual vocabulary words (Vocabulary) or determining common relationships between pairs of words (Similarities). Stronger scores in these areas often suggest adequate verbal concept development. He also had little difficulty responding to *"why"* types of questions about social rules and regulations (Comprehension). Jeremy performed less competently when responding to questions pertaining to general knowledge of facts and events (Information), suggesting mild difficulty with long-term memory and retrieval skills. A relative weakness was observed on tasks requiring short-term memory skills, such as when repeating digits heard aloud (Digit Span) or solving arithmetic problems in his head (Arithmetic). Jeremy especially had difficulty repeating digits in reversed order, indicating weak active working memory skills as well.

Jeremy's nonverbal problem solving skills were slightly more sophisticated than his overall verbal abilities. He performed well when arranging blocks (Block Design) and assembling puzzles (Object Assembly) to form various designs, indicating good visual-spatial and logical problem solving skills. His overall visual attention to detailed information (Picture Completion) was sound as well. Jeremy demonstrated little difficulty in his ability to sequence *"mixed up"* pictures in order to tell a meaningful story (Picture Arrangement), suggesting an adequate knowledge of cause and effect relationships. A mild weakness was observed on a paper and pencil task requiring him to copy various symbols when timed (Coding). Lower scores on this measure often indicate limited active working memory skills, as well as slower visual-motor speed. *Jeremy's overall profile of scores indicated average general problem solving skills, with weaknesses noted on tasks involving active working memory skills, and visual-motor speed.*

**VISUAL-MOTOR PROCESSING:** On the **VMI**, a test of visual-motor integration skills requiring students to copy various geometric designs, Jeremy scored **97**, which was in the **Average** range of functioning, and at the **42nd** percentile compared to peers. This score indicated little difficulty with visual-motor integration skills. Jeremy exhibited a strong left-handed dominance throughout the evaluation, and tended to hold his pencil perfectly straight when working. Still, he tended to work in a slow and cautious manner, constructing the images in an awkward inside to outside manner. In fact, he frequently attempted to rotate his paper, though he was restrained from doing so. Often, students with difficulty in visual-motor integration tend to struggle on most paper and pencil tasks, copying information from the board, and may have difficulty with visual/spatial aspects of reading and math.

**PHONOLOGICAL PROCESSING:** The Comprehensive Test of Phonological Processing (C-TOPP) was administered in order to assess Jeremy's ability to blend and segment sounds, his phonological memory skills, and his ability to rapidly name objects from memory. Tests of phonological awareness as well as rapid naming skills tend to be excellent measures of pre-reading skills, as well as good predictors of future reading success. The following scores were obtained:

| composite | score | percentile | Range |
|---|---|---|---|
| Phonological Awareness | 67 | 1% | Impaired |
| Phonological Memory | 73 | 3% | Borderline |
| Rapid Naming | 82 | 12% | Low Average |

Jeremy's overall profile of scores suggested he lacked many prerequisite skills in order for adequate reading development to commence. For instance, he had difficulty identifying and segmenting syllables in words (i.e. say the word "*snail*" without "*n*"), as well as when asked to repeat back sounds backwards (phoneme reversals). There were also limitations noted with his short-term memory skills for sounds as well. Lower scores in these areas suggest poor phonological awareness skills, difficulty sequencing sounds, and limited working memory skills. Jeremy also exhibited mild difficulty when asked to name letters, numbers, and objects rapidly in an accurate manner. Lower scores in these areas usually indicate a slower rate of visual/verbal retrieval skills, and indicate the potential for future reading and written language difficulty.

**ACADEMIC MEASURES:** The ***Wechsler Individual Achievement Test (WIAT)*** is an individually administered test of academic achievement assessing Reading, Math, Listening, and Written Language skills. This test was co-normed with the Wechsler Intelligence Scales, thus all standard scores have a mean of *100*, and standard deviation of *15*, indicating *68* percent of students score between *85* and *115*. The following scores were obtained:

| SUBTEST | SS | GRADE EQUIV |
|---|---|---|
| Basic Reading | 67 | K.8 |
| Spelling | 69 | 1.6 |
| Reading Comprehension | 64 | 1.4 |
| Written Expression | 71 | K.0 |
| **Broad Reading** | **62** | **1.3** |
| **Broad Written Language** | **64** | **K.0** |

**READING:** Jeremy exhibited overall reading skills at an approximately  *1*ˢᵗ grade level, and at the $1^{st}$ percentile compared to peers. He exhibited extreme difficulty with his phonemic awareness skills, and was unable to blend multiple sounds to identify words. Jeremy had a tendency to misread letters, such as a "*b*" for a "*d*", and did not possess much automaticity with his sight-word recognition skills. The process of reading seemed quite taxing for him, and he was unable to utilize context clues to determine meaning from print. His overall passage comprehension skills were also on an approximately $1^{st}$ grade level.

**WRITTEN LANGUAGE:** Jeremy's ability to provide written responses to a variety of questions requiring knowledge of spelling, punctuation, capitalization, and word usage was on approximately a **kindergarten** level, and at the $1^{st}$ percentile compared to peers. He attempted to spell words in a phonemic manner, though he often was able to identify only the initial sound. A written language sample revealed that he was unable to construct a complete sentence and had extreme difficulty spelling words in a phonetically consistent manner. His written output was brief, and filled with severe grammatical and spelling errors that interfered with comprehension.

**ACADEMIC SUMMARY:** *Jeremy appeared to have a mixed subtype of dysgraphia, as well as a mixed subtype of dyslexia. This was demonstrated by multiple perceptual and lexical difficulties pertaining to the reading and written language process. Both disorders are characterized by a combination of phonological errors when reading and spelling and limited active working memory skills, in addition to orthographic errors depicting faulty sequential arrangement of letters.*

**WORKING MEMORY:** Various subtests were administered from both traditional neuropsychological measures in addition to components from contemporary memory batteries. From the Halstead-Reitan neuropsychological test battery, Jeremy was administered the **Trailmaking Test A**, a visual spatial task that required him to connect a series of 15 dots. His overall time of **20 seconds** was an adequate score. **Trailmaking Test B** is a similar measure, but this time Jeremy was required to alternate between numbers and letters while connecting dots. This task requires more attention and concentration as well as good working memory skills. His time of **99 seconds** was somewhat slow and suggested very limited working memory skills, a necessary requirement when shifting from letters to numbers.

The **Sequences** subtest was administered from the **Children's Memory Scales** in order to assess his overall active working memory skills more comprehensively. This subtest required Jeremy to sequence auditory information such as the days of the week or months of the year as quickly as possible. He demonstrated extreme difficulty on this measure, scoring in the **Impaired** range and at the *1ˢᵗ* percentile compared to peers. Jeremy often lost his train of thought while working and seemed easily distracted on this measure. He exhibited a tendency to rehearse the information verbally (subvocalization) in order to refresh his memory before decay occurred.

From the **Woodcock-Johnson III**, the **Auditory Working Memory** subtest was administered in order to assess his working memory skills more comprehensively. He was presented with a list of animals or foods, interspersed with numbers, and asked to sequence the items in the same order in which they were presented. His overall standard score was **75**, which was in the **Borderline** range of functioning, and at the **5ᵗʰ** percentile when compared to peers. Jeremy demonstrated extreme difficulty recalling items in a particular sequence and often was unable to recall the individual words in their correct order. He performed somewhat better when recalling numbers in their correct order. Once again, active working memory is defined as the amount of cognitive workspace needed to perform a given task. Often, students with deficits in written language possess limited active working memory skills, due to the simultaneous memory demands of writing. It should be noted that Jeremy also exhibited difficulty repeating back numbers in reversed order from the WISC III (Digit Span), suggesting limited active working memory skills as well.

*WORKING MEMORY SUMMARY: Jeremy exhibited significant working memory deficits, which refers to the ability to store information temporarily while simultaneously performing another task. This may have profound classroom implications. For instance, he may have difficulty recalling the beginning of a sentence while reading words at the end, as well as "visualizing" and manipulating symbolic representations needed to assist with spelling and math skills. In addition, most students with dysgraphia possess limited working memory skills, as the written language process tends to require too many simultaneous memory recall skills to be executed effectively.*

*RETRIEVAL FLUENCY SKILLS:* The *Verbal Fluency* subtest from the **NEPSY**, a developmental neuropsychological instrument, was administered in order to determine specific processing deficits that may be hindering Jeremy's ability to read and write. Jeremy had extreme difficulty retrieving words using phonemic cues, though he performed much better when retrieving words by semantic cues. For instance, he was able to name categories of items rapidly, such as animals or foods *(16/minute)*, but was unable to name items rapidly that started with the letter "*f*" or "*s*" *(3/minute)*. This suggested significant deficits with phonological storage and retrieval.

In addition, the **Retrieval Fluency** subtest from the **Woodcock-Johnson III** was administered to determine how many items Jeremy was able to retrieve from memory in a minute. His overall standard score of **90** was in the **Average** range of functioning, and at the **25**th percentile compared to peers. Once again, this task required Jeremy to use semantic cues, not phonological cues, to retrieve information in a rapid fashion from memory.

*RETRIEVAL FLUENCY SUMMARY: Jeremy exhibited difficulty with phonological processing and retrieval skills, a task usually mediated by left temporal lobe functioning. In other words, he struggled with word retrieval skills when relying upon phonological cues because he was unable to access language very effectively. Conversely, he had little difficulty utilizing semantic cues to retrieve items from memory. This type of learning profile suggested Jeremy tended to categorize information in a singular fashion - namely, by semantics - and that he may rely solely on these cues when attempting to identify words in print. Furthermore, a great deal of research indicates that students who have not grasped sound/symbol correspondence by age 12 may never acquire this skill, and need to rely on alternative strategies to develop effective reading and spelling skills.*

*EXECUTIVE FUNCTIONS:* The **Behavior Rating Inventory of Executive Functioning (BRIEF)** was administered to determine if Jeremy's difficulty with attention in school was interfering with more global behaviors such as organization skills, emotional self-control, goal directed behavior, and working memory skills. All of these cognitive processes, sometimes termed executive functions, play a vital role in the ability to plan and executive any goal directed, problem-solving task. A T-score of **65** or higher represents a significant score. Using Jeremy's parents as the respondents, the following scores were obtained:

## SUMMARY

| Behavior Rating Scale of Executive Functions (BRIEF) | | | |
|---|---|---|---|
| scale/index | T-score | percentile | average |
| **Inhibit** – Assesses the ability to resist an impulse and to stop one's own behavior at the appropriate time. | 69 | 96% | Sig |
| **Shift** – Assesses the ability to move freely from one situation to another as the circumstances demand. A key aspect of shifting includes the ability to change focus from one mindset or topic to another. | 74 | 98% | Sig |
| **Emotional Control** – Assesses a child's ability to modulate emotional responses. | 76 | 98% | Sig |
| **Behavioral Regulation Index** – Represents a child's ability to modulate emotions and behavior via appropriate inhibitory control. | 76 | 97% | Sig |
| **Initiate** – Assesses behaviors relating to beginning a task or activity. | 66 | 93% | Sig |
| **Working Memory** – Measures the capacity to hold information in mind for the purpose of completing a task. Working memory is essential to carry out multistep activities, complete mental arithmetic, or follow complex instructions. | 80 | 99% | Sig |
| **Plan/Organize** – Measures the child's ability to manage future-oriented task demands. | 80 | 99% | Sig |
| **Organization of Materials** – Measures orderliness of work, play, and storage spaces. | 71 | 99% | Sig |
| **Monitor Assesses work** – checking habits and whether a child keeps track of the effect their behavior on others. | 78 | 99% | Sig |

| scale/index | t-score | percentile | average |
|---|---|---|---|
| **Metacognition Index** – Represents the child's ability to self manage a given task. | 81 | 99% | Sig |
| **Global Executive Composite** – A summary score that incorporates all eight clinical scales of the BRIEF. | 81 | 99% | Avg |

Jeremy's overall *Global Executive Composite* score was *81*, which was in the *Extremely Significant* range of functioning, and at the *99th* percentile compared to peers. This score suggested extreme difficulty regulating his behavior and organizing his thoughts in order for successful learning to take place. There were numerous concerns in the *Metacognition Index*, as Jeremy was described as having difficulty beginning homework assignments, often making careless errors, becoming easily distracted, and often underestimating the time required to finish most tasks. There were also concerns with *working memory*, meaning that Jeremy often lost his place or train of thought while working, tended to forget multiple step directions, had difficulty concentrating, and often needed adult supervision to complete most routine tasks. In other words, Jeremy had extreme difficulty monitoring his own behavior and thought processes while engaged in a task, and thus was prone to many careless errors. In addition, there were concerns expressed regarding his difficulty with organization skills and ability to plan a task.

His parents also noted numerous concerns in the *Behavior Regulation Index*, as Jeremy was reported as being easily frustrated and having poor emotional self-control. For instance, he apparently tended to overreact to small problems, was prone to angry outbursts, and was often overwhelmed by longer assignments. There were additional concerns expressed regarding his ability to work toward a desired goal, due in part to his propensity for intense outbursts and tendency to frustrate quickly.

*SUMMARY AND RECOMMENDATIONS:* Jeremy is a 10-year-old student currently in the 5th grade at Hunt Valley Elementary School. He was referred for a neuropsychological evaluation due to continued difficulty acquiring basic reading and written language skills in addition to a persistent pattern of intractable learning problems. He has been receiving special education services in addition to speech and language therapy since 2nd grade. Still, he was reported as making minimal educational progress, despite numerous intervention strategies, most of which centered on explicit phonics instruction. Current testing indicated Jeremy's overall cognitive abilities were in the lower end of the **Average** range of functioning **(FSIQ=91)**, with his nonverbal problem solving skills being slightly more developed than his verbal abilities. Jeremy's overall profile of scores indicated average general problem solving skills, with weaknesses noted on tasks involving active working memory skills and visual motor speed.

In terms of his academic achievement, Jeremy's overall reading and written language skills were severely impaired, and on approximately a **beginning 1st** grade level. Jeremy exhibited limited independent reading skills and tended to make whole word substitution errors based upon the initial letter detected. This type of error pattern suggested an extremely limited phonological base, as Jeremy tended to over-rely on the visual contour and shapes of words to elicit his best guess. However, his overall sight word recognition skills were extremely limited as well, as he lacked specific strategies to assist with word identification skills. Interestingly, he tended to use both his left and right hand to track words on the page while reading. In summary, Jeremy demonstrated numerous signs of having **mixed dyslexia** in addition to a **mixed subtype of dysgraphia**. He demonstrated multiple perceptual and lexical difficulties pertaining to the written language process, characterized by a combination of phonological errors when spelling in addition to orthographic errors depicting faulty sequential arrangement of letters.

From a neuropsychological perspective, Jeremy exhibited three specific factors suggesting difficulty accessing the left hemisphere (normally the dominant hemisphere for both reading and writing) when engaged in most academic tasks. First, Jeremy was somewhat late in developing a hand dominance, thus prompting the school to force him to choose a preferred hand for writing. Though Jeremy writes left-handed, he performs many other tasks right-handed or often alternates between hands. Interestingly, both biological parents were right-handed, leaving just a 2 percent chance that he should become left-handed. One possible explanation is that Jeremy is a **pathological left-hander**, meaning he was biologically destined to become right-handed as well but was forced to switch dominance on certain activities due to some early developmental insult to the left-hemisphere. Once again, the left hemisphere is the region of the brain that modulates motor output on the right side of the body as well as right-handedness. Handedness is often a powerful indicator of the brain's dominant language centers as well. Thus, Jeremy was almost forced to become left-handed to subserve a skill normally assumed by an intact left hemisphere.

Second, despite years of explicit phonics training, Jeremy possessed virtually no phonemic awareness skills, and had extreme difficulty retrieving words using phonics cues as well as with most rapid naming tasks. The ability to identify words through phonemic analysis, a foundation skill necessary for further reading to commence, is performed only by the left hemisphere, not the right. Lower scores on rapid naming tasks often indicate a slower rate of visual/verbal retrieval skills, as well as the potential for future reading difficulty. In essence, Jeremy's reading may reflect his right hemisphere's attempt to modulate a task for which it was not designed.

Jeremy also displayed extreme difficulty with **working memory skills** (the amount of memory needed to complete a given cognitive task) in addition to significant **executive function deficits**. Active working memory refers to the ability to store information temporarily while performing another task simultaneously. Thus, he may exhibit difficulty recalling the beginning of a sentence while reading words at the end, as well as *"visualizing"* and manipulating symbolic representations needed to assist with spelling and math skills. Working memory also plays a vital role in the storage of information into long-term memory.

Lastly, Jeremy was rated as having limitations with **executive functioning**, which refers to an array of skills such as sustaining his attention, planning and organizing, following a sequence of steps, and self-monitoring task performance. Perhaps no other academic skill requires more planning and organization than written language, which was his greatest academic deficit. Though much research has identified the left frontal lobe as modulating many of these skills, the entire brain plays a role in the execution of many of these tasks. Given this scenario, the following recommendations are offered:

## READING RECOMMENDATIONS:

1. It is recommended that explicit phonics instructional approaches be discontinued in teaching Jeremy to read. His neurodevelopmental profile suggested he may never acquire basic sound/symbol associations to use as a foundation for further reading skills.

2. Jeremy may benefit from a modified **Language Experience** approach to reading. For instance, the teacher might ask him to dictate a story about a topic of high interest, then read back his story from dictation. Based upon his reading errors, the teacher then would create color-coded pictorial word-cards where the word is outlined and a picture drawn next to the word. The word-cards would eventually be presented in isolation, without the outlined perimeter around the word and the picture.

3. Jeremy may benefit from the **Neurological Impress** method of teaching reading. This involves using high interest reading materials in the following manner:

> (a) Have the teacher initially read a passage while Jeremy follows along.
> (b) Jeremy and his teacher engage in co-joined reading of the passage together, while his teacher uses her finger to rapidly track each word.
> (c) Have Jeremy read the passage separately using his finger to track the words.
> (d) Create word-cards for reading miscues.

4. Jeremy may benefit from specific computer software programs assisting in reading. The **Henderson** program, which involves using semantic cues to identify words, may be especially helpful. In addition, Jeremy may benefit in the future from the **Lexia** program, which is more of a phonics-based program but may be useful once he establishes a greater base of sight words.

## CLASSROOM RECOMMENDATIONS:

5. Jeremy would benefit from having most books on tape as well as recordings from more lecture-oriented courses.

6. Jeremy would benefit from being allowed to dictate most written classroom assignments.

7. Jeremy may benefit from taking tests and quizzes in his special education classroom to help eliminate distractions.

8. Classroom modifications such as preferential seating in the front of the room, working with a *"study buddy"* to double-check work, and using subtle refocusing cues such as a light touch on the shoulder may be helpful for him. Also, Jeremy should be asked to repeat directions verbally in order to ensure comprehension.

## MEMORY RECOMMENDATIONS:

9. Given Jeremy's limitations with working memory, he may benefit from verbal rehearsal strategies (e.g., talking cues) to keep information in memory for a longer time. Teaching him to *"talk"* his way through multi-step or multi-sequential tasks, such as division, may be helpful as well. Also, reading aloud as opposed to silently may assist with comprehension.

10. Jeremy might learn and remember best through experiential learning, such as field trips, science activities, or role-playing events, as opposed to listening to verbal instructions.

11. Jeremy's teachers and parents should work together to develop an organizational notebook that will enable Jeremy to function more efficiently both at school and at home. Consultation with the school psychologist is recommended.

12. Jeremy may perform better with multiple choice tests and recognition tests as opposed to exams with questions that require free recall.

## WRITTEN LANGUAGE RECOMMENDATIONS:

13. The use of flashcards and computer software that promote visual recognition might be beneficial for Jeremy's spelling skills. The ***cover-write*** method, which provides kinesthetic feedback through large-muscle movement, might be an effective strategy to assist with spelling as well.

14. Jeremy may benefit from learning keyboarding skills so he can effectively operate a computer and word processor to assist with written language assignments.

15. Provide Jeremy with sentence combining activities in order to strengthen syntactical structures of written expression. Present word sequences out of order, and ask him to construct whole sentences from combinations of the words. Next, present sets of phrases that must be properly sequenced to create more complex sentences, then finally whole sentences to be constructed into paragraphs.

16. Jeremy may benefit from computer software instructional approaches to writing to assist him in recognizing the patterns of language, from letter shapes to word spellings to sentence structures. For instance, the ***CAST Universal Design for Learning*** computerized instructional system is centered on pattern recognition skills and strategic functioning skills, and emphasizes internal drive and motivation.

# Remediation Strategies for Dysgraphia

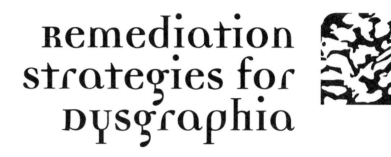

# Chapter 10

*"You tell me, and I forget; you teach me, and I remember; you involve me, and I learn."*
— Benjamin Franklin

A colleague was invited to conduct a series of seminars on neuropsychological assessment in the aftermath of the Chernobyl incident in the former Soviet Union. Scores of innocent townspeople had been exposed to harmful radiation emanating from a Soviet power plant following an unprecedented explosion. As the former Soviet government tried in vain to diminish the public perception of the magnitude of the disaster, it became apparent that many survivors as well as individuals in neighboring towns were suffering from subtle, and often not so subtle, learning and language deficits. Soon the demand for neuropsychological assessment intensified as thousands of innocent Russians were demonstrating *soft signs* of mild brain impairment. Consequently, American psychologists established a series of training seminars for Russian psychologists to discuss the utility of neuropsychological assessment. The primary goal was to enhance the overall proficiency with which Russian psychologists were assessing language, memory, cognition, and other higher-level cortical skills that may have been impaired in the incident. During the course of the seminars, the discussion turned away from individual diagnostic procedures and data analysis toward more specific remediation techniques. As expected, a fundamental question with which most neuropsychologists wrestle was eventually raised - namely, at what point should interventions be directed toward rectifying a specific weakness such as poor memory or word retrieval skills, versus utilizing remaining strengths to override the apparent weakness? In other words, is the brain capable of retraining itself when assisted by a specific remediation technique, or should interventions be geared toward forging new neural pathways to accomplish a particular cognitive task?

The response from Russian psychologists to the American trainers was somewhat surprising, though upon closer inspection rather predictable due to the vast differences between the two cultures. In the Soviet perception, Western civilization is often viewed as a pop-culture market driven by a rugged sense of invincibility, overt optimism, and need for immediate gratification. Hence, the philosophical orientation toward remediation approaches in the Western world remains the "*quick fix*" mentality, laced with pre-packaged intervention approaches to tackle virtually any cognitive dysfunction. In fact, our educational system is often driven by the notion of a *magic bullet* paradigm, as most educators spend countless hours searching for an aesthetically perfect teaching strategy to correct learning difficulties. This mentality was somewhat maligned by the Soviet psychologists, who viewed the entire concept of remediation through a different prism, one which reflected the hardships and tribulations of their economically impoverished society. More conservative and less Pollyannish in their efforts, the Soviets viewed human cognitive functioning as a highly complex phenomena resulting from the expression of an infinite array of neuronal activity. Given the brain's 100 trillion or so connections among its 100 billion neurons, they considered the entire notion of a simplistic teaching alteration or structured learning exercise leading to a formidable cure somewhat foolish. The fact of the matter was that subtle neurological deficits were not "*fixed*", as if repairing the transmission of an automobile, but rather were accepted as a more permanent limitation. Therefore, the goal of remediation was more compensatory in nature, focusing on strengthening preserved functions as opposed to retraining specific impairments.

Rather than political predispositions or cultural differences dictating the course of interventions for cognitive dysfunction, the science side of psychology - namely *clinical neuropsychology* - can serve as the beacon of light harboring insights and truths regarding human abilities and disabilities. Discarded is the notion of "*one size fits all*" that often preys upon the American education system, leading to a homogeneous classroom model for all children. Instead, specific remediation strategies need to be tailored to the individual learner based upon the neurodevelopmental strengths and weaknesses of the child coupled with the maturation of the brain. The fundamental premise guiding specific remediation strategies is the notion that mental stimulation during early childhood activates brain cells for processing new information and setting down memories. It is during this critical period, and especially during the first three years of life, that the foundations for thinking, language, vision, attitudes, aptitudes, and a host of other characteristics are laid down in the basic wiring of our brains. Then the windows in the brain slowly begin to close, and much of the fundamental architecture is completed (Kotulak, 1997). Therefore, the key to actually re-routing and re-teaching brain cells to perform a given cognitive task is early intervention, before specific brain regions become fully mature or *myelinated*. Once a neural network has been established, support cells begin to surround the network of axons and the myelination process begins (Kolb & Whishaw, 1996). The myelination of various brain regions begins in infancy and continues into adulthood, and signals the full maturity or *"hard wiring"* of certain brain regions. Hence, there are certain windows of opportunity for learning based upon the developing nervous system, brain growth spurts, and subsequent myelination process. Table 10-1 summarizes the most opportune time for learning:

## TABLE 10-1

| The Timing of Learning | | |
|---|---|---|
| AGE | SKILL | BRAIN REGION |
| 3 -10 months | Attention & Awareness | Reticular Formation |
| 2 - 4 years | Language Acquisition | Temporal Lobes |
| 6 - 8 years | Phonemic Development | Inferior Parietal and Temporal Lobes |
| 10 - 12 years | Abstract Language | Inferior Parietal Lobes and Frontal Lobes |
| 14 - 16 years | Judgement & Planning | Frontal Lobes |

* Increment in brain weight 5-10 percent over each 2-year period
* Expansion not due to neuronal proliferation, but rather growth in dendritic processes and myelination.

Perhaps no other neurological concept has had a more profound effect on teachers and parents than the knowledge that sensory experience is essential for teaching brain cells their jobs, and that after a certain critical period, brain cells lose the opportunity to perform these jobs (Ramachandran, 1998). For example, if the brain does not process visual experiences by age two, the capacity will be lost, and if a child is not exposed to language by the age of 10, the person will never acquire this skill (Kotulak, 1997). Therefore, the key to educating the brain lies in the ability to stimulate and enrich certain brain regions at critical junctures in the developing nervous system. With respect to dysgraphia, the most essential remediation strategy lies not in a particular written language program, learning series, or educational methodology, but rather in the *matching* of a particular program, series, or educational strategy with an individual learner's neurodevelopmental profile.

### *Language-Based Interventions:*

Over one-third of the words in a standard English dictionary have more than one pronunciation; more than fifty percent of these contain silent letters; and most letters, especially vowels, have more than one sound (Clark & Uhry, 1995). Our schools have systematically attempted the harrowing task of teaching correct spelling by assigning weekly spelling words followed by a quiz. Since most academic calendars follow a 36-week school year, and the average number of spelling words assigned each week is approximately 15, most students have been quizzed on some 3,240 words between 1st through 6th grade. Since the average 5th grader begins to encounter some 10,000 new words each year, with printed English containing some 85,000 distinct word families, it is inconceivable that one can teach spelling through the painstaking analysis of drill and practice of each and every word. According to Levine (1999), spelling should be assessed within the context of written expression. In other words, standardized spelling lists may provide some indication of whether or not a student is on grade level, but performance is often based upon the number of words spelled correctly as opposed to the difficulty of the word. Furthermore, most parents and teachers often lament that students may spell a word correctly on an individual spelling test but spell the same word incorrectly in the context of a sentence. Therefore, a careful analysis of a child's misspellings should reveal persistent error patterns that need to be targeted by prudent educators. In any event, the following approaches were designed to assist with spelling disorders within the contextual framework of written expression.

***Alphabetic Phonics:*** This is an expansion of the Orton-Gillingham multisensory approach for teaching reading to children with dyslexia. This program has been revised numerous times since its inception in the mid 1960's. The program assumes that 80 percent of the 30,000 most commonly used English words can be considered phonetically regular and therefore predictable once the basic rules have been learned (Clark, & Uhry, 1995). Based on Samuel Orton's theories, this program uses visual, auditory, and kinesthetic activities to develop a coding pattern for the English language. Progress is documented through benchmark measures that examine letter knowledge, alphabetizing skills, reading, spelling, and handwriting. The structured daily lesson takes an hour to complete, with 11 different activities lasting approximately 5 minutes long. This is an explicit (synthetic) type of phonics approach, as letter-sound correspondences are taught in a *"bottom-up"* fashion before whole words are introduced. The program is designed for children from elementary school through high school, and there are numerous alpha-phonics teacher-training centers throughout the United States.

Despite the widespread inclusion of multisensory techniques in remedial programs for students with dyslexia and dysgraphia, and the almost unanimous conviction among practitioners that they work, there is little empirical data to validate their effectiveness (Clark & Uhry, 1995). If anything, multisensory techniques appear to vary instructional activities and minimize boredom. There are many variations of the alphabetic phonics program, and the program is flexible enough to focus on emerging reading and written language skills for elementary students and more advanced stages of reading comprehension and written language skills for secondary students. Perhaps the most efficient use of **Alphabetic Phonics** occurs with students with phonological subtypes of dysgraphia and dyslexia.

**Making Words:** The purpose of this procedure is to help students develop basic phonemic awareness skills and discover how the alphabetic system works by increasing their understanding of sound-letter relationships. This strategy is geared toward younger students and can be used along with regular writing activities (Cunningham & Cunningham, 1992). *Making words* activities begin with relatively short words and ultimately build toward longer words utilizing all of the letters. Children manipulate the letters to produce a variety of words. Each activity takes approximately 15 minutes. Emphasis in all activities is placed on how words change when letters are moved and different letters are added. The following steps are used:

1. Provide each student with 6-8 letters that they use to make 12 to 15 words.
2. Ask each student to make two-letter words using all of the letters.
3. Ask each student to make three-letter words using all of the letters.

4. Continue the pattern, increasing word length by one letter during each step. The final word, a six-, seven-, or eight-letter word, will include all of the letters the student has for that day.

***Writing to Read:*** This program was designed as a beginning reading program for students in kindergarten and 1st grade using a combination of cooperative learning, small group instruction, and cooperative learning centers (Clark & Uhry, 1995). The fundamental premise of the program is that children will learn to read words they have composed more efficiently than words from another source. *Writing to Read* assumes that children enter school knowing approximately 2000 words that they are capable of combining in syntactically appropriate ways. The goal is for children to apply their pre-existing syntactical knowledge of words towards writing combinations of letter sounds in words, which allows them to grasp the alphabetic principle. There are six work centers including:

1. *Computer Center* - 42 phonemes are introduced sound by sound within the context of 30 words.
2. *Writing/Typing Center* - children are encouraged to type words and edit their work.
3. *Activity Center* - hand-form letters are practiced using tactile materials such as clay or sand utilizing a multi-sensory approach.
4. *Work Journal* - students listen to an audio tape and practice writing by hand as well as reinforce rhyming skills.
5. *Make Words* - materials such as plastic letters are used to assemble words.
6. *Tapes Library* - 23 books available to listen using an audio cassette.

One advantage to the *Writing to Read* program is that teachers can be trained relatively quickly through in-service workshops, and there are no rigid scripts to be followed. In essence, this program combines computer technology with multisensory stimulation to promote both reading and writing proficiency among younger students in a phonemic manner.

***Cover-Write Method:*** Perhaps more than any other cognitive skill, written language requires the harmonious synchronization of multiple perceptual and lexical processes, thus placing undue emphasis on the ability to retrieve information effectively into active working memory. For individuals who experience difficulty in retrieving word images (which is often the case in **surface dysgraphia**), the *cover-write* method may be useful. It involves air tracing as a means of assisting students in retrieving word images. The concept of air tracing does not produce a distinct visual image, but does provide kinesthetic feedback through large-muscle movement. The following procedure, described by Kirk and Chalfant (1984), consists of several steps:

1. Select a word for the student to learn, then write the word on a card and pronounce it.
2. Next, have the student pronounce the word.
3. Have the student look at the word and say the letter names or sounds while tracing each letter in the air.
4. Remove the word and have the student pronounce the word while tracing it in the air.
5. If necessary, repeat step 3.
6. Have the student continue pronouncing the word while tracing it in the air until the spelling is known.
7. Have the student pronounce the word while writing it on paper. If the word is spelled incorrectly, repeat step 3.
8. Follow the same steps to teach a new word.
9. Have the student write the word in a notebook that can be used for review purposes.

**Fernald Method:** The Fernald method also helps the student to develop a visual image of the word and to spell the word accurately (Mather & Roberts, 1995). Pronouncing a word while simultaneously forming a visual image can be an effective study technique for students who have difficulty recalling the orthographic representations of words, such as in **surface dysgraphia**. The technique (a) draws attention to the word, (b) provides an auditory-visual link, and (c) controls the direction of word inspection. The following steps are used:

1. Have the student select the word to be studied.
2. Write the selected word on a piece of paper.
3. Have the student repeat the correct pronunciation while looking at the word.
4. Provide the student with time to develop a visual image of the word. Place emphasis upon humor to draw up a unique visual image of the word that can be remembered.
5. When the word has been learned, have the student write the word from memory.
6. If the word is written incorrectly, return to step 3. If the word is written correctly, have the student turn the paper over and write the word another

time from memory.

7. Create opportunities for the student to use words in writing sentences.

**Visual Spelling:** As noted in Chapter 6, working memory involves the ability to hold representational knowledge of the environment in mind coupled with the mental flexibility to manipulate this knowledge in whatever manner one chooses. A key component of our working memory store is visual imagery. The ability to visualize information in the mind's eye is vital for the memorization of specific letter formations, spelling patterns, and punctuation rules. Some students have difficulty sequencing sounds but have good recall of visual images. Other students may excel with phonological processing skills but struggle with visual recall. For those students, spelling phonetically irregular words may be especially difficult, and thus they may benefit from the technique described by Glazzard (1982). The following steps are incorporated in this method:

1. Write a sentence on the board including the spelling word in context.
2. Construct a drawing of the word underneath the word itself.
3.  Read the sentence aloud with the student.
4. Erase the picture and the word.
5. Ask the student to read the sentence, verbally adding the correct (pictured) word in the blank.
6. Write the correct spelling of the pictured object in the blank, spelling the word aloud while writing it.
7. Have the student read the sentence aloud once again.
8. Give the student a copy of the sentence with the spelling word on the line and a drawing of the word under the line.
9. Have the student copy the spelling word at the front of the sentence, verbalizing the sounds as the word is spelled.
10. Repeat the procedure for all the spelling words.

**Musical Spelling:** Some students, particularly those with multiple perceptual deficits, may particularly benefit from more nontraditional instructional techniques. Martin (1983) recommended combining spelling practice with music to assist students with severe spelling deficits. This method has proven particularly successful with individuals who have experienced failure and frustration with spelling in the past due to a combination of poor phonological processing and visual-spatial limitations. After all, music allows for the classification of sounds using rhythm, pitch, melody, and timbre. The phonological aspect of spelling also involves a sound classification system - namely, the alphabetic code, which is primarily modulated by the left temporal lobe. Even though melodies tend to activate the right temporal lobe, music often evokes such strong emotional responses that it serves as sort of an acoustical beacon capable of being linked to specific memory schemas and facilitating recall of personal events. According to Levine (1999), this type of paired association learning, which links spelling to music, is often more desirable than learning by drill and repetition. Hence, a unique approach to learning and recalling spelling is forged by using one sound classification system (music) to trigger another (alphabetic code). Such multisensory approaches to vocabulary building might include looking at a word, pronouncing it, tracing it, then picturing it by way of a visual image while a particular song is playing. The following steps may be used for increasing spelling awareness:

1. Review the spelling words and their meanings with the student.
2. Write down the words and their meanings.
3. Have the student review the first two words.
4. Have the student record the first two words on a tape recorder by:
   a. spelling the first word
   b. pronouncing the word
   c. defining the word
   d. following steps a through c with the second word
1. Repeat step 4 while a tape of a favorite song is playing.
2. Turn off the two tapes while the student reviews the next two words.
3. Have the student repeat steps 4-6 until all the spelling words have been recorded.
4. Ask the student to listen to the tape every morning and evening until the day of the test.

***Language Experience Approach:*** The language experience approach (LEA) can be combined with several strategies such as semantic mapping in order to improve writing skills (Mather & Roberts, 1995). The basic procedure of the LEA involves these steps:

1. Have the student share an experience.
2. Write or type the ideas as the student dictates a story about the experience.
3. Have the student read the story back.

Kaderavek and Mandlebaum (1993) describe several teaching strategies that can be used to foster idea development during the oral discussion stage of LEA. Throughout this process, modeling techniques and questioning strategies should be used to increase student involvement and promote writing skills. The following steps are included:

1. Construct a semantic map as students describe an experience.
2. In the middle of the map, write a word critical to the experience.
3. Brainstorm on different words and arrange them in categories around the topic.
4. After the map has been developed, have students dictate a story about the experience into a tape recorder.
5. Ask each student to evaluate and critique the clarity, organization, and specificity of each part of the story. In addition, students can decide what type of story frame or text structure is best suited to their narrative.
6. Have students discuss the organization of their narrative, then dictate their story a second time.
7. Have the students write the dictated story.
8. Have the students read the story aloud.

***CAST Universal Design for Learning:*** In the **UDL** computerized model, it is assumed that students must recognize the patterns of language, deploy expressive language strategies, and possess a strong amount of persistence in order to become successful writers. The instructional system is based on a rudimentary understanding of brain functioning, but it is refreshing in its attempts to correlate specific instruction with the neurodevelopmental profile of the child. The specific brain functions driving the program are centered on pattern recognition skills, strategic functioning skills, and internal drive and motivation. For instance, difficulties with spelling, grammatical conventions, and composition instruction all fall within the pattern recognition skills section. On the other hand, difficulties with penmanship, planning, and organization fall within the purview of the strategic function section. Lastly, poor self-esteem, low expectation of success, and difficulty sustaining effort throughout the written language process fall under the internal drive and motivation section. The program stresses the development of classroom environments that promote flexibility in instruction and support individual differences between learners. In addition, it emphasizes a multisensory format for instruction with software that allows students to record spoken ideas digitally and play them back, draw images or diagrams, or enter text. Also, students can change the size, color, or font of the text to highlight certain features. Therefore, through color, animation, and interactivity, computers can help emphasize and isolate patterns as well as provide opportunities to practice and explore through active manipulation of words and text (Meyer et. al., 2001). For further information regarding the UDL system, contact http://www.cast.org.

***Writing Skills for the Adolescent:*** This program primarily focuses on the augmentation of the handwriting, spelling, and composition skills of students who are both dysgraphic and dyslexic. Developed by Diane King, this training program was designed for use in conjunction with traditional Orton-Gillingham reading instruction and based on its fundamental principles. Included is a multisensory approach for teaching reading and written language to children with an educational disability. Based on Samuel Orton's theories, this program uses visual, auditory, and kinesthetic activities to develop a coding pattern for the English language. Progress is documented through benchmark measures, examining letter knowledge, alphabetizing skills, reading, spelling, and handwriting.

The ***Writing Skills for the Adolescent*** program features a "*bottom-up*" type of approach, since free writing without the necessary prerequisite skills is discouraged so poor habits will not be reinforced. The curriculum begins by asking students to write single words, then sentences, paragraphs, and essays. A key component of the ***Writing Skills for the Adolescent*** program is the continued emphasis on grammar. Grammar is taught by requiring students to compose sentences rather than completing workbook exercises, and involves progression from parts of speech to various types of clauses. In addition, there are exercises designed for *logical thinking* skills, allowing students to compose topic sentences as well as devise techniques for weaving sentences together in a coherent and logical order. From a neuropsychological perspective, the breadth of this program allows for remediation of virtually any type of dysgraphia, though it may be especially helpful for semantic/syntactic dysgraphia. Given the emphasis on ordering thoughts and ideas logically into a fluid paragraph, students with executive functioning deficits as well as difficulty with working memory skills may benefit as well.

***Sentence combining:*** Sentence-combining activities have become increasingly popular among speech and language therapists who wish to increase syntactic maturity in students. There are many versions and variations, though to begin, students are asked to write two or three smaller sentences that are then combined into a longer, more elaborate sentence. All suggestions are discussed and all acceptable sentences produced by students are written on the board. If desired, exercises may focus on a specific aspect of syntax, though emphasis should be placed on instruction in a variety of sentence patterns. A sentence-combining strategy, adapted from Nutter and Safran (1984), suggests adherence to the following steps:

1. Construct simple sentences in one of two ways:
   a. Compose from the student's spelling and vocabulary words.

    b.  Deconstruct sentences from the student's textbooks.

1. Teach any unfamiliar words out of context.
2. Provide oral practice with the sentences before asking the student to combine them in writing.
3. Guide and provide encouragement when the student attempts written work.
4. Supply any requested spellings.
5. Accept all answers that are grammatically correct.
6. Encourage creativity, not just correctness.
7. Use the strategy several times per week for 5 to 15 minutes.

**Step Up to Writing: (Sopris West):** This technique uses color-coding to enable students to visualize and structure words into meaningful sentences and paragraphs. Using the colors of a traffic signal, students are taught to see which aspects of their writing skill needs improvement. For instance, the color green means "*go*", and students are asked to choose the information they want to share on a given topic. The color yellow means "*slow down*" and students must select key concepts and phrases to support their topic sentence. Finally, the color red means "*stop*" and students must stop and present evidence and ideas to support their passage. Lastly, the color green emerges again as students are reminded to go back and restate the topic. Using colored strips of paper, students learn to write down their thoughts one time, then organize and prioritize their sentences into paragraphs using color-coded traffic signs. Lesson plans are geared toward all grade levels.

Training is an integral component to the *Step Up to Writing* program, with the most common approach being a four-day, 30-hour training seminar. However, shorter seminars are available as well, with follow-up programs recommended for teachers to maximize their success with individual students. The *Step Up to Writing* program is one of the few comprehensive and systematic written language programs geared toward children of all grade levels, and should be especially helpful for students who struggle with semantic/syntactic dysgraphia.

**Sentence Writing Strategy:** A subcomponent of the University of Kansas' Strategic Instruction Model, this program consists of two primary parts, the *Fundamentals in the Sentence Writing Strategy and Proficiency in the Sentence Writing Strategy*. Both involve strategies that allow students to recognize and write 14 sentence patterns consisting of simple, compound, complex, and compound-complex sentences. All of the strategies have been field-tested with students who have been judged to have learning disabilities. The instructor's manual features a systematic sequence of instructional procedures.

Also included within this framework is the ***paragraph writing strategy***, which helps students organize and plan ideas related to a topic, develop a sequence of ideas to be expressed, and structure verb tenses within a paragraph. The ***error monitoring strategy*** assists students with proofreading written work for content as well as mechanical errors. For further information regarding these sets of instructional materials or information regarding instructor training, contact *The University of Kansas Center for Research on Learning* at www.ku-crl.org.

***COPS Strategy:*** One of the most salient features of effective writing skills is the ability to plan and develop an idea in an organized fashion within a particular narrative style. Most skilled writers tend to compose a *rough draft* first, then fine-tune their written product through a painstaking set of procedures known as *rewrites*. This approach to writing trains the brain to execute a variety of self monitoring functions including spell-checks, grammar checks, punctuation checks, and checks for general content and clarity. For those students who struggle with executive functioning types of skills and lack the strategic know-how to evaluate the quality of their work accurately, the following strategies may be helpful:

**C** **CAPITALIZATION** - Check capitalization of first words in sentences and proper nouns.
**O** **OVERALL** appearance of work - Check for neatness, legibility, margins, indentation of paragraphs, and complete sentences.
**P** **PUNCTUATION** - Check commas and end punctuation.
**S** **SPELLING** - Check to see if the words are spelled correctly.

***SCAN Strategy:*** The mnemonic SCAN (Graham & Harris, 1987) can be used to help students clarify sentences. The letters represent the following steps:

**S** Does the sentence make *sense?*
**C** Is the sentence *connected* to my beliefs?
**A** Can more be *added?*
**N** Have I *noted* all the errors?

***SCOPE Strategy:*** This strategy, described by Bos and Vaughn (1994), is similar to the COPS strategy. Its primary purpose is to foster and develop more efficient proofreading skills. The strategy consists of the following series of questions that the student applies to writing:
**S** Is the *spelling* correct?

**C** Are the first words, proper names, and nouns *capitalized*?

**O** Is the syntax or word *order* correct?

**P** Are there *punctuation* marks where needed?

**E** Does the sentence *express* a complete thought?

  Does the sentence contain a noun and a verb?

**C-SPACE:** Some students benefit from having a mnemonic to help them remember specific strategies. The mnemonic C-SPACE (MacArthur et al., 1991) may be used as a prewriting strategy. Prior to writing, ask the student to decide (a) for whom the story is being written and (b) what kind of story they want to write. Next, have the student take notes on the story, using the following mnemonic:

**C** Who is the *character*?

**S** What is the *setting*?

**P** What is the *problem* or purpose?

**A** What *action* occurs?

**C** What is the *conclusion*?

**E** What is the *emotion* of the character?

**POWER:** This is a process oriented approach to written language based on the notion that children with learning disabilities have significant difficulty analyzing text structure and are relatively poor at self-monitoring the writing steps. This technique is especially useful for students who lack the meta-cognitive skills to monitor elements of the writing process such as syntax, spelling, grammar, and intended audience. It is intended either for regular classrooms or special education resource rooms serving children with learning disabilities. The acronym POWER emphasizes the following steps:

*Plan* - students are encouraged to consider their audience and the purpose for the assignment, and take into account their own background knowledge of the topic.

*Organize* - involves categorizing and sequencing ideas.

*Write* - the first draft is constructed on colored paper, saving white paper for final revision.

*Edit* - think sheets are used to self-edit, as well as a peer review

*Revise* - putting check marks next to editing corrections.

According to Englert (1990), the POWER steps must be supported by dialogue during the writing process by having the teacher *think aloud* the various steps. In addition, graduated prompts are used by the teacher to guide students through each step, and eventually the prompts are replaced by students utilizing *self-talk* to coach themselves through the process.

***Story Maps:*** Graphic organizers can also be used to help students develop story maps for writing (Mather & Roberts, 1995). Teachers may want to incorporate the following procedures for utilizing story maps into narrative writing:

1. Choose an appropriate story map for a writing assignment.
2. Draw the map on the chalkboard.
3. Explain the purpose and benefits of using story maps.
4. Brainstorm organizational ideas with students.
5. Give students a blank copy of the map and have them copy from the board.
6. Assist students in synthesizing information to create a story.
7. Provide less detailed maps until students can organize them individually.

***Writing Wheels:*** Writing wheels (Rooney, 1990) can also be used to help students who experience difficulty with executive functioning domains. This method assists students to develop their ability to organize essays, paragraphs, compositions, or term papers. The wheels are used to separate the main ideas and details. Each wheel is produced on a separate page, and the writer then adds details, ideas, and thoughts in a spoke-like fashion around the wheel. When all the ideas have been recorded, the writer numbers the ideas in the sequence in which they will be presented. For instance:

1. Write the title at the top of the paper.
2. Draw five wheels on the first sheet. In the first wheel write the word START and in the last wheel write the word END. Write a word or phrase or sentence in the first wheel that identifies the ideas that will be used in the introduction.
3. Write one main idea inside each of the three middle wheels that will be developed.
4. In the last wheel, marked END, write a word, phrase, or sentence that will be used as the conclusion.

## TABLE 10-2

| summary of Language-Based Intervention techniques | |
|---|---|
| Phonological Dysgraphia: | Alphabetic Phonics<br>Making Words<br>Writing to Read |
| Surface Dysgraphia: | Cover-Write Method<br>Fernald Method<br>Visual Spelling |
| Mixed Dysgraphia: | Musical Spelling<br>Language Experience Approach<br>CAST: Universal Design for Learning<br>Software programs (Table 10-3) |
| Semantic/Syntactic Dysgraphia: | Writing Skills for the Adolescent<br>Sentence Combining<br>CAST; Universal Design for Learning<br>Step Up to Writing (Sopris West)<br>Sentence Writing Strategy (University of Kansas)<br>Software Programs (Appendix 10-3) |
| Executive Functioning Deficits: | COPS<br>SCAN<br>SCOPE<br>C-SPACE<br>POWER |
| Working Memory Deficits: | Graphic Organizers<br>Story Maps<br>Writing Wheels |

Steven G. Feifer, Ed.S., NCSP   Philip A. De Fina, Ph.D., ABPdN

## TABLE 10-3

### computer software instructional program

#### computer software

**ACTA.** Scottsdale, AZ: Symmetry.

**AppleWorks.** Santa Clara, CA: Claris.

**AppleWorks GS.** Santa Clara, CA: Claris.

**Bank Street Writer III.** New York, NY: Scholastic Software.

**Bank Street Writer Plus.** Novato, CA: Broderbund Software.

**Beamer: Prefixes, Basewords, Suffixes.** Kanakee, IL: Data Command.

**Big Book Makers.** Calabasas, CA: Toucan.

**Bilingual Writing Center.** Fremond, CA: The Learning Company.

**Capitalization (Grades 3-9).** Diamondale, MI: Hartley.

**Capitalization (Grades 5-12).** Big Springs, TX: Gamco.

**Cause & Effect.** Campton, NM: Troll.

**Children's Writing and Publishing Center (English or Spanish).** Fremont, CA: The Learning Company.

**Complete Spelling Program.** Minneapolis, MN: SLED Software.

**Create with Garfield.** Blacklick, OH: Science Research Associates.

**Disney Comic Strip Maker.** Northbrook, IL: Mindscape.

**Dr. Peet's Talking Text Writer.** Diamondale, MI: Hartley Courseware.

**Easy Report Writer.** State College, PA: Parrot Software.

**Easybook.** Center Harbor, NH: Chickadee.

**English on the Job.** Omro, IL: Conover.

**Essential Grammer.** Big Springs, TX: Gamco.

**Essential Punctuation.** Big Springs, TX: Gamco.

**FrED Writer.** Concord, CA: Cue SoftSwap.

**Grammer Baseball.** Big Springs, TX: Gamco.

**Great Beginnings.** Gainesville, FL: Teacher Support.

**Grolier Writer.** Boston, MA: Houghton Mifflin.

**Homonyms, Antonyms, and Synonyms.** Big Springs, TX: Gamco.

**How to Write for Everyday Living.** Long Island, NY: Educational Activities.

**IBM Process Writing Package.** Atlanta, GA: IBM Educational Systems.

**Keyboarding Primer.** St. Paul, MN: MECC.

**Keytalk, Audio Word Processor.** Calabasas, CA: PEAL Software.

**Kids and Keys.** Fairfield, CT: Spinnaker.

**Kidsworks II.** Torrance, CA: Davidson & Associates.

**Kidwriter.** Fairfield, CT: Spinnaker.

**Kidwriter Golden Edition.** Fairfield, CT: Spinnaker.

**Language Activities Courseware.** Boston, MA: Houghton Mifflin.

**Language Arts.** Boston, MA: Houghton Mifflin.

**Language Experience Recorder Plus.** Gainesville, FL: Teacher Support.

**Little Riddles.** Diamondale, MI: Hartley.

**Logo Express.** Montreal, Canada: Logo Computer Systems.

**Logo Writer.** Montreal, Canada: Logo Computer Systems.

**Lucky Seven Spelling Games.** Fairfield, CT: Queue.

**Lucky Seven Vocabulary Games.** Fairfield, CT: Queue.

**MacWrite.** Santa Clara, CA: Claris.

**MacWrite II.** Santa Clara, CA: Claris.

**MacWrite Pro.** Santa Clara, CA: Claris.

**Magic Slate.** Pleasantville, NY: Sunburst.

**Magic Spells.** Fremont, CA: The Learning Company.

**Make-A-Book.** Gainesville, FL: Teacher Support.

**Mavis Deacon Teaches Typing.** Chicago, IL: Mindscape.

**Microsoft Works.** Bellevue, WA: Microsoft.

**MicroType: Wonderful World of Paws.** Florence, KY: Southwestern.

**Mind Reader.** Campbell, CA: Brown Bag Software.

**Monsters and Make-Believe.** Calabasas, CA: Toucan.

**Muppet Slate.** Pleasantville, NY: Sunburst.

**My Own Stories.** St. Paul, MN: MECC.

**My Words.** Diamondale, MI: Hartley Courseware.

**New Print Shop.** Novato, CA: Broderbund Software.

**Newsroom.** Fairfield, CT: Spinnaker.

**Once Upon a Time.** New Haven, CT: CompuTeach.

**101 Misused Words.** Lake Zurich, IL: Learning Seed.

**Outliner.** St. Paul, MN: MECC.

**Printshop.** Novato, CA: Broderbund.

**Punctuation Baseball.** Big Springs, TX: Gamco.

**Punctuation Rules.** Norfolk, CT: Optimum Resource.

**Read, Write, and Publish Series.** Acton, MA: William K. Bradford.

**Sensible Grammer.** Troy, MI: Sensible Software.

**Sensible Speller.** Troy, MI: Sensible Software.

**Sentence Starters.** Gainesville, FL: Teacher Support.

**Sound Sentences.** Long Island, NY: Educational Activities.

**Special Writer Coach.** Cambridge, MA: Tom Snyder.

**Spell It Plus.** Torrance, CA. Davidson & Association.

**Spelling Mastery.** Blacklick, OH: Science Research Associates.

**Spelling Puzzler.** Boston, MA: Houghton Mifflin.

**Spelling Puzzles and Tests.** Minneapolis, MN: MECC.

**Spelling Rules.** Norfolk, CT: Optimum Resource.

**Spelling Speechware (1-6).** Boston, MA: Houghton Mifflin.

**Spelling Tutor.** Houston, TX: Access Unlimited.

**Spelling To Be Somebody.** North Billerica, MA: Curriculum Associate.

**Spellright Software.** North Billerica, MA: Curriculum Associates.

**Spider Hunt Spelling.** Big Springs, TX: Gamco.

**Stickybear Parts of Speech.** Norfolk, CT: Optimum Resource.

**Stickybear Spellgrabber.** Norfolk, CT: Optimum Resource.

**Stickybear Typing.** Norfolk, CT: Optimum Resource.

**Storybook Weaver.** St. Paul, MN: MECC.

**SuperPrint for the Macintosh-English.** Jefferson City, MO: Scholastic.

**SuperPrint for the Macintosh-Spanish/Bilingual.** Jefferson City, MO: Scholastic.

**Talking Text Writer.** New York, NY: Scholastic Software.

**That's My Story.** Chicago, IL: Mindscape.

**The Print Shop.** Novato, CA: Broderbund Software.

**The Student Writing Center for Windows.** Fremont, CA: The Learning Company.

**Type to Learn.** Pleasantville, NY: Sunburst.

**Typing Keys.** Novato, CA: Academic Therapy.

**Typing Tutor.** New York, NY: Scholastic Software.

**Vocabulary Builders.** Big Springs, TX: Gamco.

**Vocabulary Challenge.** Chicago, IL: Mindscape.

**Vocabulary Detective.** Pine, AZ: SWEPS Educational Software.

**Vocabulary Development.** Norfolk, CT: Optimum Resource.

**Vocabulary Machine.** Gainesville, FL: Teacher Support.

**Webster's New Word Spelling Dictionary.** Des Moines, IA: Simon and Schuster.

**Word Capture.** Tulsa, OK: Heartsoft.

**Word Launch.** Tulsa, OK: Heartsoft.

**Word Magic.** Chicago, IL: Mindscape.

**Write Now.** Lakewood, NJ: MacWarehouse.

**Write This Way.** Katonah, NY: Interactive Learning Materials.

**Write This Way-LD.** Diamondale, MI: Hartley Courseware.

**Writing Adventure.** Blacklick, OH: Science Research Associates.

**Writing Center.** Fremont, CA: The Learning Company.

**Writing to Read.** Atlanta, GA: IBM Educational Systems.

**Writing to Write.** Atlanta, GA: IBM Educational Systems.

**Writing Workshop.** St. Louis, MO: Milliken Publishing Company.

Instructional programs

Handwriting

**A Writing Manual for the Left-Handed.** Cambridge, MA: Educators Publishing Service.

**Alphabet Mastery (Letters).** Novato, CA: Ann Arbor.

**Beginning Connected, Cursive Handwriting (Levels 1-3).** Cambridge, MA: Educators Publishing Service.

**Creative Cursive.** Grand Rapids, MI: Instructional Fair.

**Cursive Writing (Letters).** Novato, CA: Ann Arbor.

**Cursive Writing (Words).** Novato, CA: Ann Arbor.

**Cursive Writing Skills.** Cambridge, MA: Educators Publishing Service.

**D'Nealian Handwriting (Cursive).** Glenview, IL: ScottForesman.

**D'Nealian Handwriting (Manuscript).** Glenview, IL: ScottForesman.

**D'Nealian Home/School Activities (Grades 1-3).** Glenview, IL: ScottForesman.

**Handwriting with Write and See.** Chicago, IL: Lyons and Carnahan.

**Handwriting without Tears.** Potomac, MD: Olsen.

**Learning to Use Cursive Handwriting.** Cambridge, MA: Educators Publishing Service.

**Learning to Use Manuscript Handwriting.** Cambridge, MA: Educators Publishing Service.

**Let's Print and Spell.** Cambridge, MA: Educators Publishing Service.

**Let's Write and Spell.** Cambridge, MA: Educators Publishing Service.

**Loops and other groups: A kinesthetic writing system.** Randolph, NJ: O.T. Ideas.

**Manuscript Alphabet.** Grand Rapids, MI: Instructional Fair.

**Manuscript Writing (Letters).** Novato, CA: Ann Arbor.

**Manuscript Writing (Words).** Novato, CA: Ann Arbor.

**Remediation of Reversals: The "Magic Rulers" Program-Revised Edition.** Novato, CA: Academic Therapy.

**Right Line Paper.** Austin, TX: PRO-ED.

**Stop-Go Right Line Paper.** Austin, TX: PRO-ED.

**The Johnson Handwriting Program.** (Cursive) Cambridge, MA: Educators Publishing Service.

**Transition to Cursive (Books 1, 2).** Grand Rapids, MI: Instructional Fair.

**Writing Exercises for the Left-Handed.** Cambridge, MA: Educators Publishing Service.

*Adapted from Mather, N. & Roberts, R., (1995). *Informal Assessment and Instruction in Written Language.* New York: John Wiley & Sons. (p. 341-342). Reprinted with permission.

# Remediation Strategies for Non-Language Dysgraphia

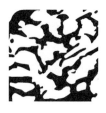

# Chapter II

*"Either write something worth reading or do something worth writing."*
*— Benjamin Franklin*

Written language is an exclusively human form of communication, requiring a highly sophisticated ability to integrate multiple cognitive capacities measured only by the direct output of a specific motor skill. Notwithstanding, linguistic, motor, visual, visual-perceptual, visual-motor, proprioceptive, kinesthetic, emotional, and cognitive functioning all need to be relatively intact and operating harmoniously under complete command of the cerebral cortex in order for successful writing to occur. The prudent examiner must always delineate between deficits falling under the purview of a language-based dysgraphia, or those belonging to a non-language or motor skill type of dysgraphia. No matter what the nature of the deficit, written language production can be regarded as a key indicator of the functional status of the human brain. The range of possible deficits that are unique to written language disorders, the specific and secondary impacts of the deficits, and the magnitude of their impact on writing remain a challenge to the child, the parents, the teachers and even the most skilled therapists. For these reasons, it is essential that those who evaluate and treat individuals with writing disorders comprehend the relationship between the brain and the diverse behaviors specific to writing.

Despite the importance of written expression for the communication of specific thoughts and ideas, the educational system tends to ignore children with dysgraphia. For instance, most remedial educational programs focus on reading deficits or enhancing mathematics prowess. Unfortunately, some students with poor written expression have been castigated as being lazy or unmotivated, while others have been relegated to more vocational aspects of the educational system. The reality of the situation is that most standardized academic tests do not focus on handwriting skills. Even accomplished teachers and experienced therapists who recognize the gravity of dysgraphia can be daunted by the apparently contradictory discussions in the salient literature. Much of this literature is based on anecdotal information or non-empirical research and experience. Furthermore, there is often a lack of commonality in the terms used and in the populations studied. Neurodevelopmental factors are often ignored. From a distance, the literature on dysgraphia can give the wrong impression of the condition it claims to depict: a lack of organization, poor prioritizing, failure to connect, irregularities, and not knowing what direction to take next. Like the dysgraphic child, therapists, teachers and parents often feel hopeless, frustrated and avoidant.

Increasingly, within school systems, occupational therapists are being called upon to work with dysgraphic children, primarily those with non-language based dysgraphia. This book has presented fundamental neuropsychological information on the relationship of the brain to writing behaviors, as well as neuropsychological research-based data that occupational therapists and other professionals can use for planning treatment as well as effective intervention strategies. For those occupational therapists fortunate enough to have an ongoing working relationship with a neuropsychologist, the groundwork for successful interdisciplinary collaboration has been laid. However, there are many occupational therapists who either lack an ongoing working relationship with a neuropsychologist or are beginning therapists and lack sufficient background experience and training to integrate neuropsychological evaluation results into the occupational therapy treatment interventions. Nonetheless, the need for systematic evaluation, diagnosis, intervention strategies, and monitoring based on a thorough understanding of a brain-based educational model of learning remains the basis for effective and efficient treatment. This chapter presents various strategies on how to integrate salient, available neuropsychological information into occupational therapy assessments and treatments of individuals with the three main non-language based dysgraphias: *ideomotor apraxia, ideational apraxia* and *constructional dyspraxia*.

In working with non-language based dysgraphia, the primary focus of assessment and intervention is on the *physical* act of constructing the written word. As mentioned previously, writing involves specific sequences of muscular actions or motor engrams. Once learned, these actions are based on specific visual and kinesthetic programs. In fact, observing the act of writing itself provides information regarding previous learning and the ability to access stored information plus current cerebral functional status. According to Sandler, et al (1992, p. 17)

*"A child's writing can be called a 'develomentogram', a record (of) the child's stylus and hand, reflecting aspects of the child's linguistic, motor and cognitive development, and adds valuable insights to the developmental neurology of information processing."*

When assessing a specific subtype of dysgraphia, the most essential component is not necessarily its categorization by name, but rather access to a theoretical framework linking specific types of behaviors with the area of the brain involved. This linkage, in turn, provides a framework for alerting the therapist regarding the other possible deficits that might be present simultaneously and the type of intervention that would be most effective. In addition, an appreciation of this brain-behavior relationship from a developmental perspective is critical in terms of planning interventions, developing strategies, and determining whether to strengthen fundamental capacities underlying the writing deficits or to focus more on developing compensatory strategies.

***Anatomical Correlates:*** Reading and writing are intricately related linguistically. Writing, however, is far more complex physiologically and neuropsychologically. While reading emanates from the external environment, writing starts from the central nervous system of an individual. The execution of a conscious motor act such as writing begins with the *precentral* motor strip. In addition, the *supplemental motor area* is involved in sequencing or planning of sequential movements as well as changes in the speed of the movement. Additional involvement from the *globus pallidus* provides information on posture and the position of the head, body and limbs. Of course, the *cerebellum* is involved in the coordination of motor skills and in visual tracking. It is also necessary to assure the smooth execution of planned movements in terms of direction, force and accuracy. The *basal ganglia* is responsible for more automatic movements. Connolly (1998) associates the cadence of writing to the basal ganglia. The integration of all these components entails prefrontal executive functions of organizing, planning, and personal choices that reflect content. Though written language involves the precentral motor strip, its smooth execution is dependent on multiple fundamental capacities located throughout the brain.

As noted previously, Goldberg (1989) argued quite poignantly that novel tasks tend to be mediated by right hemispheric functioning, while skilled, over-learned tasks tend to be modulated by left hemispheric functioning. Therefore, learning new motor acts such as letter formation skills are initially mediated by the right cerebral hemisphere, though once learned, the skilled act of writing is housed in the left hemisphere. By skilled, we refer to those movements involving complex, sequenced components that are practiced, learned, and automated as an aggregated entity. Individual components that comprise skilled movements are grouped, stored, and recalled as an *engram* (Luria, A. 1980; Brown, & Minns, R.A. 1998).

Motor act engrams can be referred to as a *motor language*, and an engram as the motor equivalent to concept formation in the cognitive domain. Different behaviors are stored in different parts of the cortex, with motor acts being stored in the motor association area and motor-hearing acts being stored in Broca's area. Significant research (Blakemore & Cooper, 1970, Blakemore, 1974, Merzernich et al, 1983) has demonstrated that early and frequent usage is capable of changing the size of the cortical representation of a specific body part in the somatosensory cortex, suggesting that maturational development of neural connections depends on usage. In other words, early manipulation and practice of fine motor skills involving paper and pencil tasks lay the cortical foundation for subsequentmotor engrams to be carried over toward the complex task of written language.

This implies that the young, developing, pre-writing child with incipient, nascent dysgraphia is establishing or learning the precursor acts and fundamental capabilities of writing in an inefficient and somewhat inappropriate way. Consequently, these ill-formed motor acts will be the bases for the engrams developed later and will be utilized in writing endeavors. In contrast, the child with acquired dysgraphia presents a selective loss in the ability to utilize previously learned motor engrams when writing, the particulars of which depend on the developmental stage of the child and the extent and location of injury. In any case, effective remediation must take into consideration the fact that the child must unlearn old fixed patterns and establish the means for new neural pathways. Since children often attempt to adapt to their deficiencies in meeting the demands of their daily lives by using their available strengths to compensate, it is important to note how they have adapted to such tasks as writing in school.

Since written language entails the integration of many language and motor based skills and abilities, a multi-disciplinary evaluation integrating sound neuropsychological knowledge in conjunction with the application of relevant principles in occupational therapy remains the gold standard for effective treatment. In order to combine neuropsychological and occupational therapy approaches regarding dysgraphia, a brief review of the three types of non-language based dysgraphias presented in Chapter 5 along with other concomitant related deficits frequently present will be discussed. This theoretical foundation will underlie targeted intervention approaches as well as therapeutic goals and objectives. There will also be a discussion regarding several selected commercial tests that can be adopted or adapted for assessment or therapeutic interventions. Once again, this discussion is limited to non-language based dysgraphia that involves a selective loss in either the ability to learn or apply fine motor skills, even though the hand is otherwise intact in terms of power and reflexes.

## TABLE II-I

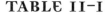

| neurological determinants of writing |
| --- |

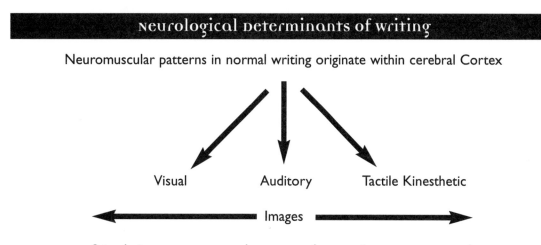

Neuromuscular patterns in normal writing originate within cerebral Cortex

Visual        Auditory        Tactile Kinesthetic

Images

Stimulating motor areas where manuel-motor images are aroused.

Conveyed to writing hand through a delicate blend of
visual - auditory - tactile - kinesthetic - linguistic processes

***Review of Subtypes:*** The defining characteristic of ***ideomotor apraxia*** is the inability to carry out a motor act on command despite being able to perform the same act spontaneously. Ideomotor apraxia involves movements that involve a single action and not sequences of actions. For example, picking up a pencil, closing a window, or touching your nose are single action movements. Children with ideomotor apraxia can perform these movements spontaneously but not on command. Ideomotor apraxia involves the left pre-motor cortex and parietal regions as well, which are the cortical areas responsible for directing the motor cortex to execute a specific movement. (See Figure 5-2). It should be noted that ideomotor dysgraphia can also involve the *arcuate fasciculus*, which mediates the necessary proprioceptive feedback between Wernicke's Area and Broca's Area.

The salient sign of *ideational apraxia* involves individuals who cannot carry out a sequence of actions, though they remain perfectly capable of doing each component action individually and on command. Concomitant to the inability to sequence, these children evidence great difficulty prioritizing, organizing, and completing multi-stepped tasks in a timely fashion. This inability indicates both temporal and spatial organizational difficulties. For these students, writing is slow and laborious. Because of proprioceptive deficits, the child fails to have adequate feedback clues, resulting in writing that is full of errors and characterized by variations in size, slant and directionality. This type of dysgraphia is associated with lesions or dysfunction of Exner's area in the left dorsolateral frontal lobe.

The hallmark of *constructional dyspraxia* is the inability to synthesize written materials visually, resulting in poor handwriting skills that stem not from motor programming but from poor spatial constraints. Deficits in the ability to synthesize visually are evidenced by poor consistency, inability to copy accurately, inability to center on the page, and difficulties in sequencing letters and words in a straight line. Deletions or duplications of letters and strokes are typical of this writing (Cubelli & Lupi, 1999). In addition, constructional dyspraxia suffers from brevity, often is mechanistic, and lacks emotional tone and creativity. The major brain regions associated with constructional dyspraxia involve dysfunctions to the right parietal lobe. However, sloppy written output can also be influenced by other factors, including working memory, especially along the visual spatial sketchpad, a temporary storage place to hold visual, spatial, and kinesthetic information as a mental image.

Within the educational system, students tend to be referred most often for occupational therapy evaluations by teachers who have noted some motor problems, including poor hand writing skills. These students evidence a number of motoric movement deficiencies that affect writing, such as poor posture while seated at a desk, poor grasp of writing utensils, inability to write in a straight line or within a given space, and difficulty completing assignments in a timely manner. In order to establish an effective remediation program, the occupational therapist must assess the appropriate developmental stage of the child's postural/muscular status, the functional status of the sensory systems (in particular, sight, auditory, tactile and proprioception), visual-motor coordination including the rhythm and cadence of movements, and visual-perceptual skills. The neurobehavioral implications of the specific subtype of motor dysgraphia must be considered as well. As always, a neuropsychological assessment provides the basic neurobehavioral profile that can be used as the cornerstone for a coordinated interdisciplinary set of interventions. In addition, the occupational therapist should review any available past reports from teachers and parents to determine where the child is functioning developmentally, prior social and medical history, and the current strengths and deficits.

***Assessment Issues for Occupational Therapists:*** The occupational therapist can begin their assessment by observing the child in the classroom or by asking the child to complete a simple writing or drawing sample. The therapist should pay particular attention to the various motor patterns used by the child, as well as whether they are rigidly repeated or evidence dynamic adaptability. The writing sample itself provides information. For instance, the Ayres Handwriting Speed Test is a good example of a standardized test for handwriting. It assesses directionality, spacing, and formation of letters. However, the test is limited to those students who have letter recognition. The following example of this test illustrates a student with constructional dyspraxia.

## FIGURE 11-1

### Ayers Handwriting speed Test

Four score and seven years ago our fathers brought forth upon this continent a new nation conceived in liberty and dedicated to the proposition that all men are created equal. Now we are engaged in a great civil war testing whether that nation or any nation so conceived and so dedicated can long endure. We are met on a great battlefield of that war.

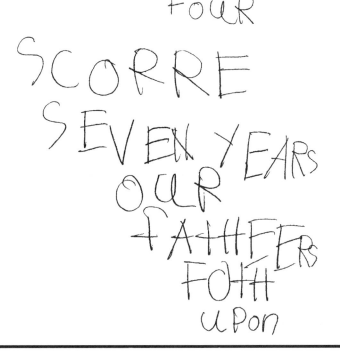

One of the most basic foundations of the development and maintenance of good handwriting skills is a dynamic, fluid, and appropriate posture. This is dependent on the integration of a number of complex sensory and motor systems that include feedback and feed-forward informational loops. A basic rule familiar to most occupational therapists states that proximal stability determines more distal stability, and must be considered of primal importance in evaluating and planning effective interventions for the dysgraphic child. A stable trunk, shoulder, and pelvic girdle provide internal stability for the necessary arm and hand mobility in writing letters sequentially. Thus, it is imperative for the child to learn the correct motor patterns that underlie writing by first learning the correct foundational postural patterns inherent to a stable trunk and shoulder girdle. Trunk, shoulder, and girdle stability can be viewed as the effectiveness of the arm in transporting the hand during a writing task and maintaining it during any necessary manipulation. Without this stability, a spiraling effect ensues: the elbow is unstable, the forearm pronates, and the metacarpal phalangeal joints lock into position and fail to move in a coordinated but individuated dissociated pattern. This is often demonstrated by a *"locking posture"* or immature grip. The child then has difficulty in achieving the necessary hand mobility for shaping written letters while moving forward rhythmically in the appropriate given space. Good handwriting also requires adequate external support; without it, the child goes into a flexed posture and becomes easily fatigued. In summary, both internal and external support must be sufficient to enable neck and head stability for visual tracking and hand-eye coordination concomitant to keeping the arm and hand free for writing.

Postural and muscular control of the trunk, pelvic, and shoulder girdle can be evaluated in a number of ways. The child can be observed rolling over, crawling, creeping, standing, and walking on terrain of graduated difficulty. Proprioceptive capacities can be observed in static and shifting of balance while sitting, standing, and walking as well as asking the child to mimic the therapist's movements, ensuring that both left and right sides are tested. It is critical to observe the student's postural control while performing school related activities, for example, in art, sports, physical education, or music groups. Obviously, functional muscle strength and tone must be assessed in all four extremities and in different positions. It is almost a truism to point out that normally maturing patterns depend upon neuromotor readiness (Gesell & Armatruda, 1969) although recent research suggests that environmental factors play a significant role. Together, these muscular actions provide the basis for neurobehavioral self-regulation, first in postural sets and then generalizing to gross motor movements, and finally to the more demanding, versatile, fine motor movements inherent in handwriting. The interrelationship between postural trunk control and writing can be observed in those children who have difficulty navigating through school halls, as they also evidence similar problems in attempting to produce the necessary motor movements inherent in written production. Rather than constructing and spacing words neatly on worksheets, these children often write to the edge of the paper with the words trailing or curving across the lines.

To assess posture and large, gross muscle patterns, there are a number of commercially available tools such as *Bruinicks Osteresky Testing (BOT)* or *Quick Neurological Screening Test-II (QNST-II)* that provide age-equivalent scores. The BOT is a standardized test that assesses gross and fine motor skills, upper extremity response speed, and dexterity. However, the BOT is not suitable for students who cannot follow specific, standardized directions within specified time lines. The QNST-II screens for neurological immaturity and impairments that may impact on the motor movements and accuracy involved in handwriting. The QNST-II, unlike the BOT, permits the modeling of the task, and its scores provide a broad baseline and level for the magnitude of neurological dysfunction. Hand strength, also necessary for writing, can be evaluated formally or informally. A dynamometer can measure grip strength formally to determine a baseline of weight resistance. Informally, the student is asked to open and close different types of containers, stretch rubbers over different shaped objects, or perform other manipulative activities involving finger and hand strength.

Fine motor skills should also be assessed to determine the age appropriate equivalent for object manipulation, coordination, dexterity, strength, endurance and motor speed for hand activities. Weaknesses in any of these skills may result in poor control of the writing utensil, fatigue, and limited persistence. The response speed and other subtests of the *Bruinicks Osteresky Testing (BOT)*, the *Minnesota Rate of Manipulation (MRM)*, the *Purdue Peg Board (PPB)*, or *ETCH* can be used to assess fine motor skills and how quickly the child can accomplish gross grasping and directionality (left/right) in tasks requiring supination and pronation. Table 11-2 illustrates basic fine-motor milestones for the developing preschool age child, which subsequently lays the foundation for the emergence of proper fine motor handwriting skills.

## TABLE 11-2

| fine motor developmental milestones | |
|---|---|
| **Age** | **Milestone** |
| 24-30 month | Cuts with scissors |
| | Traces a cross |
| | Builds tower of 9 blocks |
| | Traces a square |
| | Catches a large ball |
| | Uses a hammer |
| | Moves individual fingers |
| | Preferential use of one hand |
| 3-4 year | Copies a square/a circle |
| | Imitates a cross |
| | V and H stroke |
| | Draws a man-head with one other part |
| | Prints letters |
| | Colors with direction |
| | Builds a tower of 10 blocks |
| | Cuts a straight line |
| | Cuts out a circle |
| | Builds with construction toys |
| | Ties a knot |
| 4-5 year | Snaps fingers |
| | Mature grasp |
| | Copies diagonal strokes |
| | Copies a triangle |
| | Traces a diamond strokes |
| | Draws a man with 7 parts |
| | Draw pictures |
| | Colors within the lines |
| | Prints simple words |

The occupational therapist must also assess the different sensory systems that impact on handwriting. The sense of pressure, texture, and temperature must be adequate in order to modulate feedback differences in objects' functioning as well as for safety. Deficits in proprioception or kinesthesia result in immature, poorly developed grasping patterns. Often the student compensates for visual or visual perception deficits by holding their head close to the paper as a means of visually monitoring the writing task.

Whether copying or writing, the visual system must be intact in order to monitor and track progress effectively. An eye examination should be a part of the formal assessment to determine both the visual acuity and the developmental stage of the visual system. Good visual control entails the ability to shift focus from near point to far point as well as tracking visually from different directions. Writing in English demands an understanding of the relationships between directionality in print. This capacity and its underlying mental representation must be developed to continue monitoring acceptable progression, and to learn to write correctly and efficiently.

Finally, visual-motor coordination of hand-eye movements must be assessed to determine the child's ability to assess and integrate measures of distance, time, and space in a smooth, efficient fine motor response. Without intact sensory and perceptual systems, handwriting looks sloppy with poor letter formation (Heubness, 1989). During the assessment, the occupational therapist observes and notes behaviors, constantly querying if the child switches hands, under what circumstances this occurs, and how posture and stability affect the child and the written product (Loikith & Ritter, 1989). Visual perceptual and visual motor skills may be assessed using commercial products such as the *Test of Visual Perceptual Skills, Test of Visual Motor Skills,* or the *Beery Test of Visual Motor Skills.* This test focuses on spacing within boundaries, shape recognition, directionality, and crossing the midline while coping shapes. One limitation is that the symbols can be memorized if the test is given too often or within short time frames.

While the prime focus of the occupational therapist is on the motor-sensory-perceptual aspects of motor dysgraphia, the psychological aspects cannot be ignored. Students with dysgraphia may present a wide range of behaviors that developed as a result of multiple motor skills deficits. Such behaviors are often demonstrated when the child frequently seeks assistance to complete writing tasks or simply refuses to engage in the task at hand. Motor dysgraphia represents not only physical and cognitive challenges but also psychological and behavioral challenges as well.

***Occupational Therapy Interventions:*** Once the essential assessment information is gathered from all available resources, both formal and informal (neuropsychological assessment, educational reports, developmental/psychological/social/medical history, occupational assessment and observations), the occupational therapist now must integrate the information so a coherent picture is formed that highlights the current sensory-motor status of each child as it applies to writing skills. The information should be reviewed to determine age-appropriate development. In addition, the type of dysgraphia should be delineated and the brain-behavioral relationship reviewed, as well as noting what other functional areas are affected due to extant neural deficits. In short, an analysis of which motor engrams are intact, coupled with which motor engrams are dysfunctional and under what circumstances, must now be completed. Only with this background can an effective remediation program be planned and implemented around the following four strategies and levels for interventions (Ehrhardt, 1994).

(1) Neurodevelopmental techniques that offer guided movement for the body in space to develop tone, proprioceptive and kinesthetic feedback, midline awareness, and balance can be utilized. These techniques focus on postural alignment and control, upper body control, motor output, and acquisition of hand skills initially through weight bearing and balance shift activities (Foltz, DeGangi, & Lewis, 1991). Neurodevelopmental treatment techniques focus first on postural deficits and gross motor movements. Remediation to improve strength and endurance can be implemented through push/pull resistive activities during physical education classes or within the academic classroom, either as an individual or group activity. In occupational therapy, remedial postural activities may be practiced using mobile equipment that facilitates the vestibular system. Proprioceptive and vestibular exercises that emphasize position and awareness of body parts in space must precede the introduction of activities entailing motor planning, e.g. manipulative activities. Placing the student in resistive positions or providing iterative resistive activities builds strength and endurance. As the child begins to master postural control, the occupational therapist can begin to combine postural activities with hand-eye coordination activities such as throwing objects at a series of static targets placed at different distances. This activity can evolve into changing one's visual focus of near point/far point as well as more dynamic postural changes. Levels of difficulty can be mediated by asking the child to move, introducing moving targets, or throwing to an established rhythm, thus combining time, space, and rhythm into the activity, all of which are essential for writing.

Additional modifications can be introduced by having the child play with other children in differently sized rooms, playing outdoors on uneven terrain, changing body positions on demand, changing equipment from static to dynamically moving, or from a wide to more narrow base stance. Visual perceptual components such as matching different shapes of objects thrown with their containers can be introduced. For example, the child can be asked to throw triangular beanbags into triangular containers, spontaneously or on demand. Mental flexibility and sequencing can be added to these activities by having the child copy a pattern of throws. For instance, first throw two left, then two right; or two red bags then two blue balls. An auditory, musical, and/or rhythmical component can be introduced by asking the child to throw only when high musical notes are played, while resting with low notes. A known melody can be used or the occupational therapist can sing the notes. It should be noted that asking the child to respond to spoken directions versus moving spontaneously addresses the defining characteristic of *ideomotor dysgraphia*. What is essential for success in this series of remediation activities is to establish and master the appropriate movement/postural patterns first so that the foundational engrams become relatively stable. Then, new demands can be added slowly and in small, incremental amounts. In addition, physical education classes and playground equipment can be especially conducive to these activities.

Fine motor activities can be introduced through games, crafts, or playing a musical instrument. These activities can be combined with play and structured activities that emphasize postural control and sensory awareness such as *Chime-Along, Peg-a-Plane* or *Kerplunk* to allow the child to integrate new motor based patterns correctly. In addition, there are many commercial products available, such as Mary Benbow's *Fine Motor Development Kit* and Susie Amundsen's *TRICS for Written Communication: Techniques for Rebuilding and Improving Children's School Skills*. These products are especially designed for handwriting remediation. In addition, Jayne Berry's *"Give Yourself a Hand"* provides many suggestions regarding how to integrate basic goals of occupational therapy into a classroom setting.

Countless studies (Atherson, Brenner, Lovell, March, 2000) have shown that the omission or addition of a *single* skill is not correlated with specific improvements in hand writing skills per se. Instead, a variety of techniques based upon sound neurodevelopmental techniques and multisensory approaches coupled with formal hand writing practice are recommended. Thus, the integration of one's foundational postural control is essential for proper grip and the necessary rhythm or cadence in writing. This seems to suggest a parallel between rhythm and cadence in written language similar to prosody and rhythm in spoken language. As spoken language has directionality and structure, written language also entails directionality, from top to bottom, left to right. This, in turn, is dependent on a sense of one's body, of centrality or midline, for example, which is essentially an understanding of non-verbal, spatially based relationships. When a deficit exists in this area, remediation should include basic body orientation exercises, such as Tae-Bo, yoga, dance, line ballroom dancing, or weight training.

In addition, the development of writing and fine motor activities should emphasize specific boundaries depicting natural starting and stopping points. For instance, the top left corner of the page could be marked, as well as the left and right margins. A commercially available program, *Calligraphics,* provides this type of orientation while emphasizing rhythm by practicing repetitive patterns with musical tunes of different cadences. As the child begins to master the basic patterns, new patterns are introduced slowly. Novelty can be added by changing the writing utensils from a pencil to a squiggle pen, erasable pen, or even different styles of mechanical pencils. *Calligraphics,* a commercial product, incorporates the necessary components for remediation of handwriting: mastery through practice, repetition, time and rhythm, cadence, feedback, and reinforcement. When combined with postural control and body orientation remediation, this program combines neurodevelopmental, academic, and therapeutic considerations into a remediation approach in teaching handwriting.

(2) A second major remediation focus for occupational therapists is on sensory integration. These interventions focus on sensory processing and awareness, utilizing the tactile and pressure senses through different developmental movements for planning and sequencing purposes, coordinating both sides of the body, and developing balance, hand-eye coordination, and body awareness in space. Intervention strategies should be structured for the student to explore, experience, and modulate the physicality of *"over, under, between, etc."* The child is an active participant in gaining mastery over the management of the required movements in their environment. Sensory integration approaches that emphasize tactile and pressure awareness through different developmental movements can be effective. Erhardt (1994) based her approach on the capacity of the central nervous system to process multimodal inputs through the afferent system from a variety of receptors connected to the skin, eyes, nose, ears, tongue, bones, joints, muscles, and internal organs. Motor control of the hand requires this sensory input and feedback mechanisms and loops. As a rule, kinesthetic and tactile remediation techniques are generic to improvements in letter quality and speed in formulating letters. The effectiveness of this approach may be enhanced in some children by using visual and verbal prompts as well.

(3) Spatial temporal adaptation techniques focus on changing the environment as the student participates within a given space and progress from primitive to mature developmental phases, linking strategies to skilled performances (Gilfogle, Grady, & Moore, 1990.). For example, by following the appropriate developmental stages and emphasizing whole body movement, the therapist can plan intervention strategies ranging from tunnel activities to platform or hammock swings, tire swings, balance beam or rebounder in the quadraped, kneeling, sitting, or standing positions. This approach can

be modified by changing the room arrangement, or by changing the amount or type of equipment set up in the treatment area.

(4) Fourth, auditory techniques using the rhythm and cadence of modulated music stimulate the cochlea-vestibular mechanism involved in processing spatial temporal aspects of sensory information. These techniques may facilitate the reorganization of neurobehavioral responses by linking tonal differences (high/low tones) to either time-based or space-based responses. Low tones are linked with body movement giving the sense of the body in space while high tones are linked with rhythm and the sense of time or cadence. The therapist can pick the music to address deficits delineated in the assessment, or if speed is deficient, choose the music that emphasizes speed responses. If directionality is the problem, construct the intervention using headsets that differentiate and reinforce a left ear, right ear behavioral response.

In conclusion, it is recommended that therapists first evaluate the needs of the individual child using a standardized assessment of handwriting ability whenever possible. This can be used as a base line measure by which progress can be measured. The planning of remedial interventions for handwriting deficits must be comprehensive, based on a neurobehavioral understanding, utilizing interdisciplinary-based information and incorporating the individual child's needs and interests. Therapy sessions should focus initially on the more obvious deficits in posture and neurodevelopmental delays generic to poor hand writing performance. Visual perceptual or visual motor deficits should be addressed in combination with postural activities as the child achieves some mastery in postural control. A functional approach should be adopted that employs a combination of multisensory activities (visual, auditory, tactile, proprioceptive) with formalized hand writing practice. In addition, the therapist should consider such factors as family support and home environment when implementing a treatment program. Reassessment, using the standardized protocols when possible, should be conducted on a regular basis in order to map progress and to refine the remediation approach. Table 11-3 provides a synopsis of these approaches.

## TABLE 11-3

## Interventions for Non-Language Dysgraphia

| Type | Characteristics *Defining | Brain Area Involved & Function | Goals/Focus in OT* | Examples of OT Treatment Modalities (Commercial Products) |
|---|---|---|---|---|
| Ideomotor Apraxia | *Inability to carry out a motor act on command<br><br>*Involves single action movements like letter writing<br><br>Difficulties with coordination and balancing activities<br><br>Difficulties with transitioning from one activity to another<br><br>Difficulty initiating given task | Left Pre-Motor Cortex (directs motor cortex in consciously executing a movement)<br><br>Arcuate Fasciculus (monitors feedback of proprioception)<br><br>Left parietal lobe (necessary for sequencing of motor acts) | Interrelationship between Words and actions movement<br><br>Object constancy and relationships (same/different)<br><br>Rhythmical movement patterns.<br><br>Establishment of alternative strategies to link motor acts and commands | Sorting<br>• Matching games<br>Sequencing activities (i.e. beads, objects)<br><br>Typing program<br>• Write Out Loud<br>Handwriting program<br>• Calligraphics<br>Vision wheel<br>Listening program techniques (i.e. Auditory Integrative Techniques, A.I.T) |
| Ideomotor Apraxia | Low frustration tolerance<br>*Inability to perform sequential motor acts, despite intact ability to perform individual component parts of the sequence.<br><br>Inability to organize/prioritize progression of motor action steps.<br><br>Time management issues<br><br>Time management issues<br><br>May be able to copy but done carelessly | Exner's Area Left dorsolateral frontal lobe (coordinates sequential activation of stored representations of visual motor aspects of linguistic knowledge) | Sequencing<br><br>Prioritizing & organizing, spatially/temporally<br><br>Organizational skills | Dot-to-dot activities<br>Tracing –inside/outside Patterns<br>Textured activities<br>Initially using non linguistic symbols (pictures/puzzles/symbols and manipulation of objects)<br>Drawing<br>-Right Side of the Brain<br>Typing programs<br>• Type to Learn<br>• Mavis Beacon<br>Handwriting program<br>• Benbow's Loops & Group<br>Vision wheel<br>Listening program techniques (i.e. Auditory Integrative Techniques(AIT) |

| Type | Characteristics | Brain Area Involved & function | Goals/focus in OT* | Examples of OT treatment modalities |
|------|-----------------|-------------------------------|--------------------|-----------------------------------|
| Constructional Apraxia | Breakdown of visual spatial motor synthesis of written material, i.e., letter & word production | Right parietal lobe (mediates emotional "color" of cognitive events; processing of metaphors & humor; regulation of prosody and visual-motor integration) | Parts to whole concepts | Commercial Products<br>Drawing – step by step from model.<br>Can use graph paper<br>Puzzles<br>Mazes<br>Games<br>• Target<br>• Board<br>• Card |
| | Poor handwriting skills NOT due to motor program process deficits but generic to poor spatial constraints | | Visual spatialmotor integration, with Emphasis on spatial synthesis | Tracing different size/shape objects<br>Tracing, copying and drawing pictures, numbers, etc.<br>Constructional activities<br>• Popsicle sticks<br>• Paper airplanes<br>• Flicker football |
| | Deficits in sequencing letters in straight line (writing trails off) | | Familiar/unfamiliar Rhythmical movement patterns | |
| | Lack of consistency in writing | | Response speed | Developmental Learning Materials-cubes, pegs, etc.<br>Tangrams/Tangoes<br>Number Lines<br>Drawing books<br>• Ed Emberly<br>• Lee Ames<br>• Novel/high interest<br>• Student generated<br>Typing program<br>• Inspirations.<br>Handwriting program<br>• Handwriting without Tears<br>Vision wheel<br>Listening program techniques(i.e. Auditory Integrative Techniques (AIT) |
| | Inability to center on a page | | | |
| | Poor visual motor integration | | | |
| | Mechanistic writing | | | |
| | Brevity in writing | | | |
| | Void or decreased emotional tone | | | |
| | Decreased creativity | | | |

| Steven G. Feifer, Ed.S., NCSP    Philip A. De Fina, Ph.D., ABPdN

# Appendix 1

## Developmental progressions in Handwriting

### Grade 1

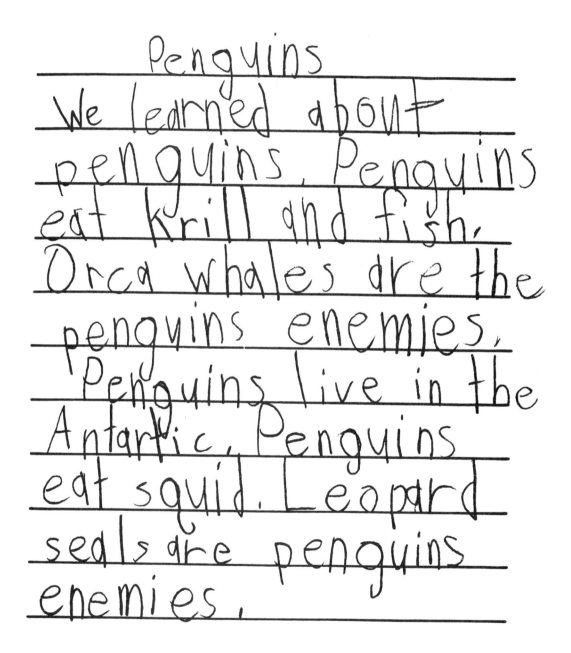

Penguins
We learned about penguins. Penguins eat krill and fish. Orca whales are the penguins enemies. Penguins live in the Antartic. Penguins eat squid. Leopard seals are penguins enemies.

Grade 2

**What is the main character's problem?  How do you know?**
**Use information from the text to support your answer.**
**(Don't forget to restate the question, give two supporting**
**details and a closing sentence.)**

Abbie's problem is that She's
scared to keep the light
on in the lighthouse, I know
this because She sowhed
scared when her dad tolled
her that She had to keep
the light on. She is allso
scared because She is scared
that her dad will not come
back to the lighthouse.
This why Abbi is scared.

| Steven G. Feifer, Ed.S., NCSP    Philip A. De Fina, Ph.D., ABPdN

Grade 3

Dear, W.WF Tribe,
These are the things we will
do at the corn festival. At my
corn festival you will weigh 1000 more
pounds more than you weigh. We'll have
very many Vegetable and we will
have turkey. My festival will have
some fighting time and some time to
pray to the corn gods. We will eat
food made out of corn. We will
play pin the tail on the turkey.
We will dress up in speacil clothes
kids will have there own place
to eat and play. We will
have the festival at harvest
and planting the festival at
planting time and narvest times. We will
chant and listen to music. We will
also dance. Those are
the things we will do at _____ Sincerly,
the festival.

grade 4

Dear Indians,
    What are you doing right now?
I invented. a new corn festival.
You can sing, dance, play, chant, make
music, and pray to the corn gods. Can
you sing this song? There was an Indians
who planted corn in Amrica. Scientists
found the corn and studied it. They
found out Indians used it, and made
it into other corn foods. They also found
out that they prayed to corn gods and
pilgrims used the corn to. When Cristor-
pher Columbus got back to Europe from
Amrica he said corn is called maize.
This corn festival is held at harvet
and planting time. There will be differen-
t games for the kids. You can make
up the games. This is all I know
about the corn fesival. and tell if me
you like this idea.                    From,

grade 5

The article about Saudi Arabia has many interesting facts. One is that Saudi Arabia is one of the few monarchies left. The current ruler is King Fahd. Another is that Saudi Arabia is a muslim nation. Saudi Arabia was the birthplace of Islam. A third fact is that Saudi people must follow strict Sahazia. In addition, Saudi women must follow even more rules. A fourth fact is that Saudi Arabia is an important country because of oil. Saudi Arabia is the World's biggest producer of petroleum. That is what I learned about Saudi Arabia.

grade 5 (gifted)

## Problem Solving Analysis

As a problem solver at the Math B level, I have specific strengths and weaknesses. When I closely examine my work, these strengths and weaknesses are evident in how well I perform in a competition. First of all, I've noticed that I gravitate towards problem solving strategies that require mainly pure mental work. I rarely use strategies where I have to map out my thinking in order to understand the problem. Though this generally works well for me, there are some problems that are written in a way that forces you to use strategies that actually do map out your thinking. Sometimes, if I come to such a problem I am stuck because I can't use or look for a pattern, work backwards, or brainstorm. If I do not balance out the strategies I use more, I will not be able to completely develop as a problem solver.

I feel that I am a fairly skilled problem solver. I get most of my answers correct and I learn much about problem solving all the time. However, I have come to acknowledge the importance of the strategies I use and have realized that I need to find a way to improve my problem solving. I've decided that rather than just start working on a problem as soon as I read it, I should carefully consider what I am being asked and think about what strategies would best fit my needs. I should also keep in mind what strategies I usually use and try to steer clear from those to keep balanced. If I do manage to keep balanced, I will expand the variety of ways that I think about problems and their solutions. I will also be able to learn more in

# REFERENCES

Alexander, M.P., Friedman, R. B., Loverso, F., & Fischer R.S., (1992). Lesion localization of phonological agraphia. *Brain and Language, 43*, 83-95.

Anderson, S.W., Saver, J., Tranel, D., & Damasio, H., (1993). Acquired agraphia caused by focal brain damage. *Acta psychologica, 82,* 193-210.

Annoni, J.M., Lemay, M.A., Pimenta, M.A, & Lecours, A., (1998). The contribution of attention mechanisms to an irregularity effect at the graphemic buffer level. *Brain and Language, 63,* 64-78.

Atherson, S., Brenner, A., & Lovell, K. (2000). *Best practices guidelines. Evidence based practice information sheet for occupational therapists.*

Baddeley, A., (2000). The episodic buffer: a new component of working memory. *Trends in cognitive science,* Nov 1; 4(11): 417-423.

Baddeley, A., (1998). Working memory. *C.R. Academy of Sciences III, 321* (2-3): 167-173.

Baddeley, A., Gathercole, S., & Popagno, C., (1998). The phonological loop as language learning device. *Psychological Review,* Jan;105(1): 158-173.

Bailet, L.L., (2001). *Development and disorders of spelling in the beginning school years.* In A.M. Bain, L.L. Bailet, & L.C. Moats *Written language disorders: Theory into practice,* (p.1) Austin, Texas, Pro-Ed Publishers.

Bain, A.M., Bailet, L.L., & Moats, L.C., (2001). *Written language disorders: Theory into practice.* Austin, Texas: Pro-Ed Publishers.

Ballator, N., Farnum, M., & Kaplan, B., (1999). *NAEP 1996 Trends in Writing: Fluency and writing conventions.* U.S. Department of Education. Office of Education And Research Improvement.

Baxter, D.M., & Warrington, E.K., (1985). Category specific phonological dysgraphia. *Neuropsychologia, 23*(5), 653-666.

Berninger, V. et al. (1997). Treatment of handwriting problems in beginning writers: Transfer from handwriting to composition. *Journal of Educational Psychology, 89,* 652-666.

Berninger, V. et al. (1998). Early intervention for spelling problems: Teaching functional spelling units of varying size with a multiple-connections framework. *Journal of Educational Psychology, 90,* 587-605.

Blakemore, C. (1974). Development of functional connections in mammalian visual system. *British Medical Bulletin, 30,* 152-157.

Blakemore , C. and Cooper, G.F. (1970). Development of the brain depends on visual experience. *Nature, 228,* 477-478.

Boice, R. (1994) *How writers journey to comfort and fluency.* Westport, CT: Praeger.

Bos, C.S. & Vaughn, S., (1994). *Strategies for teaching students with learning and behavior problems* (4th ed.). Boston: Allyn and Bacon.

Brown, J.L. and Minns, R.A.. (1998). Neurological aspects of learning disorders in children. In Whitman K., Hart. H., and Williams G. (Eds.) *A neurodevelopmental approach to specific learning disorders.* Clinics in Developmental Medicine, Number 145. London, Mac Keith).

Bruning, R. and Horn, C. (2000) Developing Motivation to Write, *Educational Psychologist,* vol. 35 (1), 25-37.

Buschke, H. & Fuld, P.A. (1974) Evaluating storage, retention and retrieval in disordered memory and learning. *Neurology* 24: 1019-1025.

Burton, A.W., & Dancisak, M.J., (2000). Grip form and graphomotor control in preschool children. *American Journal of Occupational Therapy.* 54, 9-17.

Cabeza, R. & Nyberg, L., (2000). Imaging cognition II: An empirical review of 275 PET and fMRI studies. *Journal of Cognitive Neuroscience,* 12(1), 1-47.

Calvin, W. (1996). *How Brains Think.* New York, NY: Basic Books.

Calvin, W.H., & Ojemann, G.A., (1994). *Conversations with Neil's brain: The neural nature of thought and language.* Reading, MA: Addison-Wesley Publishing Company.

Cameron, C. A., Hunt, M. K. & Linton, A. J. (1996) Written expression as recontextualization: Children write in social time. *Educational Psychology Review,* 8, 125-150.

Carroll, J.B. (1993). *Human cognitive abilities: A survey of factor-analytical studies.* New York: Cambridge University Press.

Carroll, J.B. (1995). Review of the book: *Assessment of cognitive processes: The PASS theory of intelligence. Journal of Psycheducational Assessment,* 13, 397-409.

Carter, R., (1998). *Mapping the Mind.* Berkeley: University of California Press.

Chow, T. W., & Cummings, J.L., (1999). *Frontal-subcortical circuits.* In B.L. Miller & J.L. Cummings: *The human frontal lobes: functions and disorder,* (p. 4), New York: Guilford Publications.

Clark, D.B., & Uhry, J.K., (1995). *Dyslexia: Theory & Practice of Remedial Instruction:* Baltimore: York Press.

Cleary, L.M. (1991) Affect and cognition in the writing processes of eleventh graders. *Written Communication,* 8, 473-507.

Codling, R. M. & Gambrell, L. B. (1997) *The motivation to write profile: An assessment tool for elementary teachers.* College Park: University of Maryland.

Connolly, K.J. (1998). The psychobiology of the hand. Chapter 15, O'Regan, M.,, Brown, J.K. *Neurological Disorders and Abnormal Hand Functions.* pp. 241- 263. Mac Keith Press. Distributed by Cambridge University Press. Clinics in Developmental Medicine, # 147).

Conway, T.W., Heilman, P., Rothi, L.J.G., Alexander, A.W., Adair, J., Crosson, B.A., & Heilman, K.M., (1998). Treatment of a case of phonological alexia with agaphia using the Auditory Discrimination in Depth (ADD) program. *Journal of the International Neuropsychological Society, 4*, 608-620.

Crystal, D. (1997) *The Cambridge encyclopedia of language.* Cambridge, England: Cambridge University Press.

Cubelli, R., and Lupi, G., (1999). Afferent dysgraphia and the role of vision in handwriting. *Visual Cognition,* Vol (6), 2., 113-128.

Cunningham, P.M., & Cunningham, J.W., (1992). Making words: Enhancing the invented spelling-decoding connection. *Reading Teacher, 46*, 106-115.

Damasio, A. (1994). *Descartes' Error: Emotion, Reason and the Human Brain.* New York, NY: Putnam and Sons.

Damasio, A.R., (1999). *The scientific American book of the brain.* New York: The Lyons Press.

DeFries, J.C., Olson, R.K., Pennington, B.F., and Smith, S.D. (1991). Colorado reading project: An update. In *The Reading Brain: The Biological Basis of Dyslexia,* eds. D. Duane And D. Gray. Parkton, MD: York Press.

De La Paz, S. (1999). Self-regulated strategy instruction in regular education settings: Improving outcomes for students with and without learning disabilities. *Learning Disabilities Research and Practice, 14*, 92-106.

Deuel, R.K., (1995). Developmental dysgraphia and motor skills disorders. *Journal of Child Neurology,* 10, 86-88.

Diagnostic and Statistical Manual of Mental Disorders: Fourth Edition (1994). *American Psychiatric Association:* Washington D.Cl

Englert, C.S., (1990). Unraveling the mysteries of writing through strategy intervention. In *Intervention Research in Learning Disabilities.* eds. T.E. Scruggs and B.Y.L. Wong. New York: Springer-Verlag.

Erhardt, R.P. (1994). *Developmental hand dysfunction: Theory, assessment and practice. 2nd ed.* Therapy Skill Builders. Tucson, AZ

Fedio, P., & Mirsky A.F. (1969) Selective intellectual deficits in children with temporal lobe or centrencephalic epilepsy. *Neuropsychologia, 7*, 287-300.

Feifer, S.G., & DeFina, P.D., (2000). *The Neuropsychology of Reading Disorders: Diagnosis & Intervention.* Middletown, MD: School Neuropsych Press.

Filley, C.M., (1995). *Neurobehavioral anatomy. Niwot, CO:* University Press of Colorado.

Flower, L. et al. (1990) *Reading-to-write: Exploring a Cognitive and social process.* New York: Oxford University Press.

Foltz, L. G., DeGangi, G., & Lewis, D., (1991). Physical therapy, occupational therapy and speech and language therapy. *In Children with cerebral palsy. A parents' guide.* Edited by E. Gerales. Rockville, MD: Woodbine House.

Frith, U., & Frith, C., (1983). Relationships between reading and spelling. In J.P. Kavanagh & R.L. Venezky (Eds.), *Orthography, reading, and dyslexia.* Baltimore: University Park Press.

Frostig, M., (1968). Education in children with learning disabilities. In M.R. Myklebust (Ed.) *Progress in learning disabilities.* New York: Grune & Stratton.

Gaddes, W.H., & Edgell, D., (1994). *Learning Disabilities and Brain Function: A Neuropsychological approach.* New York: Springer-Verlag Publishers.

Gardner, H. (1985). *Frames of Mind: The Theory of Multiple Intelligences.* New York: Basic Books.

Gardner, H.. (1999). *Intelligence Reframed: Multiple Intelligences for the 21st Century.* New York: Basic Books.

Gesell, A. and Armatruda, C.S. (1969). *Developmental diagnosis.* 2nd ed., revised and enlarged. New York: Harper and Brothers.

Gilfogle, E.M., Grady, A.P., & Moore, J.C. (1990). 2nd edition, Children Adapt. Thorofare, NJ. Slack Publisher

Glazzard, P. (1982). A visual spelling approach: It works. *Academic Therapy, 18,* 61-64.

Goldberg, E., (2001). *The executive brain: Frontal lobes and the civilized mind.* New York: Oxford University Press, Inc.

Goldberg. E. (1990). *Contemporary Neuropsychology and the Legacy of Luria.* New Jersey: Lawrence Erlbaum Associates, Publishers.

Goldberg, E., (1989). Gradiental Approach to neocortical functional organization. *Journal of Clinical and Experimental Neuropsychology, 11(4),* 489-517.

Goldberg, E., & Costa, L.D., (1981). Hemisphere differences in the acquisition and the use of descriptive systems. *Brain and Language, 14,* 144-173.

Goldman-Rakic, P.S., (1992). Working memory and the mind. In A.R. Damasio: *The scientific american book of the brain:* (p. 91). New York: The Lyons Press.

Graham, S. (1990) The role of production factors in learning disabled students' compositions. *Journal of Educational Psychology, 82,* 781-791.

Graham, S. & Harris, K.R. (2000) The role of self-regulation and transcription skills in writing and writing development. *Journal of Educational Psychology, v35 no. 1,* 3-13.

Graham, S., & Harris, K.R. (1987). Improving composition skills of inefficient learners with self-instructional strategy training. *Topics in Language Disorders, 7,* 68-77.

Graham, S., MacArthur, C., & Schwartz, S. (1995). Effects of goal setting and procedural facilitation on the revising behavior and writing performance of students with writing and learning problems. *Journal of Educational Psychology, 87,* 230-240.

Gregg, N., & Hafer, T., (2001). Disorders of Written Expression. In G.R. Lyon & J.M.Rumsey, *Neuroimaging: A window to the neurological foundations of learning and behavior in children:* (pp.111). Baltimore, MD: Paul H. Brookes Publishing Company.

Gubbay, S.S., & de Klerk, N.H., (1995). A study and review of developmental dysgraphia in relation to acquired dysgraphia. *Brain and Development,* 17, 1-8.

Hayes, J. R. (1996) *The science of writing.* Mahwah, NJ: Lawrence Erlbaum Associates, Inc.

Hayes, M. and Daiker, D. (1984) Using protocol analysis in evaluating responses to student writing. *Freshman English News,* 13, 1-5.

Hernstein, R.J., & Murray, C. (1994). *The Bell Curve: Intelligence and class structure in American life.* New York: Free Press.

Heubness, R., (1989). Written output "A glimpse of the total picture". *Occupational Therapy Week.* Merion Publisher, Inc.

Hillocks, G., & Smith, M.W., (1991). *Grammar and usage.* In J. Flood, J. M. Jensen, D. Lapp, & J.R. Squire (Eds.), *Handbook of research on teaching the English language arts* (pp.591-603), New York: Macmillan.

Hurford, J., Knight, C., & Studdert-Kennedy, M., (2000). *The Evolutionary Emergence of Language: Social function and the origins of linguistic form.* Cambridge University Press. p.219-230.

Hurford, D.P., Schauf, J.D., Bunce, L., Blaich, T., & Moore, K. (1994). Early identification of children at risk for reading disabilities. *Journal of Learning Disabilities,* 27 (6), 371-382.

Jarvis, P.E., & Barth, J.T., (1994). *The Halstead-Reitan neuropsychological test battery: A guide to interpretation and clinical applications.* Odessa, FL: Psychological Assessment Resources.

Jodzio, K., (1995). Neuropsychological description of memory impairment following cortical and subcortical brain injuries. *Polish Psychiatric Journal,* 29 (4),491-501.

Jones, D. and Christensen, C. (1999). The relationship between automaticity in handwriting and students' ability to generate written text. *Journal of Educational Psychology,* 91, 44-49.

Kaderavek, J.N., & Mandlebaum, L.H., (1993). Enhancement of oral language in LEA: Improving the narrative form of children with learning disabilities. *Invention in school and clinic,* 29, 18-25.

Kandel E., Lu, Y., & Hawkins, R.D. (1999). Cellular/Molecular Nitric Oxide Signaling contributes to late phase LTP and CREB Phosphorylation in the hippocampus. *Journal of Neuroscience.* The official Journal of the Society for Neuroscience. Vol. 19 (23), 10250.

Kaufman, A.S. (1994). *Intelligent Testing with the WISC III.* New York: John Wiley & Sons, Inc.

Kertesz, A., (1994). Neuropsychological evaluation of language. *Journal of Clinical Neurophysiology,* 11(2), 205-215.

Kimura, D., (1999). Sex differences in the brain. In A.R. Damasio, *The Scientific American book of the brain:* (pp.168-169). New York: The Lyons Press.

Kirk, S.A., & Chalfant, J.C., (1984). *Academic and developmental learning disabilities.* Denver: Love.

Kolb, B., & Whishaw, I.Q., (1995). *Fundamentals of Human Neuropsychology: Fourth Edition.* New York: W.H. Freeman and Company.

Kotulak, R., (1997). *Inside the Brain.* Kansas City: Andrews McMeel Publishing.

Krasuski, J., Horwitz, B. & Rumsey, J.M., (1996). A survey of functional and anatomicalneuroimaging techniques. In G.R. Lyon & J.M. Rumsey, *Neuroimaging: A window to the neurological foundations of learning and behavior in children:* (pp.25-55). Baltimore, MD: Paul H. Brookes Publishing Company.

Levine, M.D., & Reed, M., (1999). *Developmental Variation and Learning Disorders.* Massachusetts: Educators Publishing Service, Inc.

Lezak, M.D., (1995). *Neuropsychological Assessment: Third Edition.* New York: Oxford University Press.

Lockith, L., & Ritter, L. (1989). *Occupational therapy week.* Merion Publisher, Inc.

Luria, A.R., (1980). *Higher cortical functions in man.* New York: Basic Books.

Lyon, G.R. (1996). Learning Disabilities. *The Future of Children: Special education for students with learning disabilities,* Vol. 6 (1), 54-73.

Lyon, G.R. & Rumsey, J.M. (1996). *Neuroimaging: A window to the neurological foundations of learning and behavior in children.* Baltimore: Paul H. Brookes Publishing Company.

MacArthur, C.A., Schwartz, S.S., & Graham, S., (1991). A model for writing instruction: Integrating word processing and strategy instruction into a process approach to writing. *Learning Disabilities Practice,* 6, 230-236.

Martin, M., (1983). Success! Teaching spelling with music. *Academic therapy,* 18, 505-507.

Mather, N. & Roberts, R., (1995). *Informal Assessment and Instruction in Written Language.* New York: John Wiley & Sons.

Matsuo, K., Nakai, T., Kato, C., Moriya, T., Isoda, H., Takehara, Y., & Sakahara, H., (2000). Dissociation of writing processes: functional magnetic resonance imaging during writing of Japanese ideographic characters. *Cognitive Brain Research,* 9, 281-286.

McCarthy, R.A., & Warrington, E.K., (1990). *Cognitive neuropsychology: A clinical introduction.* New York: Academic Press, Inc.

McCutchen, D. (1996) A capacity theory of writing: Working memory in composition. *Educational Psychology Review*, 8, 299-325.

Meece, J. L. and Miller, S. D. (1993) Why teachers select specific literacy assignments and students' reactions to them. *Journal of Reading Behavior*, 25, 69-95.

Merzenich, M. N., & Kaas, J. H. (1982) Reorganization of mammalian somatosensory cortex following peripheral nerve injury. *Trends in Neuroscience*, 5, 434-436.

Meyer, A., Murray, E., & Bisha B., (2001) *More than words: Learning to write in the digital world.* In A.M. Bain, L.L. Bailet, & L.C. Moats *Written language disorders: Theory into practice*, (p.146) Austin, Texas, Pro-Ed Publishers.

McGrew, K.S. (1994). *Clinical Interpretation of the Woodcock-Johnson Tests of Cognitive Ability Revised.* Massachusetts: Allyn and Bacon Publishing.

Mirsky, A.F., Pascualvaca, D.M., Duncan, C.M., French, L.M., (1999). A model of attention and its relation to ADHD. *Mental Retardation and Developmental Disabilities*, 5, 169-176.

Moats, L.C. (1993). Spelling error analysis: Beyond the phonetic/dysphonetic dichotomy. *Annals of Dyslexia*, 43, 174-185.

Moro, A., Tettamanti, M., Perani, D., Donati, C., Cappa, S.F., Fazio, F., (2001). Syntax and the brain: Disentangling grammar by selective anomalies. *Neurolmage*, 13, 110-118.

Naglieri, J.A., (1999). *Essentials of CAS Assessment.* New York: John Wiley & Sons, Inc.

Nutter, N., & Safran, J., (1984). Improving writing with sentence combining exercises. *Academic therapy*, 19, 449-455.

Ogden, J., (1996). Phonological dyslexia and phonological dysgraphia following left and right hemispherectomy. *Neuropsychologia*, 34 (9), 905-918.

Ohare, A.E., & Brown, J.K., (1989). Childhood dysgraphia: An illustrated clinical classification. *Child Care Health Development*, 15(2), 79-104.

Orton, S.T., (1925). Word-blindness in school children. *Archives of neurological Psychology*, 14, 581-615.

Page-Voth, V. & Graham, S. (1999). Effects of goal setting and strategy use on the writing performance and self-efficacy of students with writing and learning problems. *Journal of Educational Psychology*, 91, 230-240.

Penniello, M.J., Lambert, J., Eustache, F., Petit-Taboue', M.C., Barre, L., Viader, F., Morin, P., Lechevalier, B., & Baron, J.C., (1995). A PET study of the Functional neuroanatomy of writing impairment in Alzheimer's disease. The Role of the left supramarginal and left angular gyri. *Brain*, 118, 697-706.

Pennington, B.F. (1995). Genetics of learning disabilities. *Journal of Child Neurology*, 10, 69-77.

Posner, M.I., & Raichle, M.E., (1994). *Images of Mind.* Oxford: W.H. Freeman and Company.

Ramachandran, V.S., & Blakeslee, S., (1998). *Phantoms in the Brain.* New York: William Morrow and Company, Inc.

Ratey, J., (2001). *A user's guide to the brain: Perception, attention, an the four theatres of the brain.* New York: Pantheon Books, Inc.

Resta, S.P., & Eliot, J., (1994). Written expression in boys with attention-deficit-disorder. *Perceptual and Motor Skills, 79,* 1131-1138.

Romani, C., Ward, J., & Olson, A., (1999). Developmental surface dysgraphia: What is the underlying cognitive impairment? *The Quarterly Journal of Experimental Psychology, 52A* (1), 97-128.

Rooney, K.J. (1990). *Independent strategies for efficient study.* Richmond, VA: J.R. Enterprises.

Sagan, C., (1996). *The demon-haunted world: Science as a candle in the dark.* New York: Ballantine Books.

Sagan, C., (1980). *Cosmos.* New York: Ballantine Books.

Sandler, A.S., Watson, T.E., Footo, M., Levine, M.D., Coleman, W.L., & Hooper, S.R., (1992). Neurodevelopmental Study of Writing Disorders in Middle Childhood. *Developmental and Behavioral Pediatrics, 13* (1), 17-23.

Sattler, J. M., (1988). *Assessment of Children.* San Diego: Jerome Sattler Publisher.

Sawyer, R., Graham, S., & Harris, K. R. (1992). Direct teaching, strategy instruction, and strategy instruction with explicit self-regulation: Effects on learning disabled students' composition skills and self-efficacy. *Journal of Educational Psychology, 84,* 340-352.

Scardamalia, M. and Bereiter, C. (1986). Written composition. In M. Wittrock (Ed.), *Handbook of Research on Teaching* (3rd ed., pp. 778-803). New York: MacMillan.

Scholz, V.H., Flaherty, A.W., Kraft, E., Keltner, J.R., Kwong, K.K., Chen, Y.I., Rosen, B.R., & Jenkins, B.G., (2000). Laterality, somatotopy, and reproducibility of the basal ganglia and motor cortex during motor tasks. *Brain Research,* Oct 6; 879 (1-2): 204-215.

Schneck, C.M., (1991). Comparison of pencil-grip patterns in first graders with food and poor handwriting skills. *American Journal of Occupational Therapy, 45,* 701-706

Schneck, C.M., & Henderson, A., (1990). Descriptive analysis of the developmental progression of grip position for pencil and crayon control in nondysfunctional children. *American Journal of Occupational Therapy, 44,* 893-900.

Schunk, D. H. and Swartz, C. W. (1993) Goals and progress feedback during reading comprehension instruction. *Contemporary Educational Psychology, 18,* 337-354.

Shaywitz, S. (1996). Dyslexia, *Scientific American, 275*(5), 2-8.

Shaywitz, S., (1998). Dyslexia. *The New England Journal of Medicine, 338* (5), 307-311.

Shell, D., et al. (1995) Self-efficacy and outcome expectancy outcomes in reading and writing performance. *Journal of Educational Psychology,* 81, 91-100.

Smits-Engelsman, B.C., & Van Galen, G.P., (1997). Dysgraphia in children: Lasting psychomotor deficiency or transient developmental delay? *Journal of Experimental Child Psychology,* 67, 164-184.

Sparrow, S., & Davis, S.M., (2000). Recent advances in the assessment of intelligence and cognition. *Journal of Child Psychology and Psychiatry,* 41(1), 117-131.

Spaulding, C. (1992) The motivation to read and write. In M. Doyle (ed.), *Reading/writing connections* (pp. 177-201). Newark, DE: International Reading Association

Strub, R.L., & Black, F.W., (1992). *Neurobehavioral disorders: A clinical approach.* Philadelphia: F.A. Davis Company.

Torgeson, J. & Hecht, S., (1996). Preventing and remediating reading disabilities: Instructional variables that make a difference for special students. In M.F. Graves, P. Van Den Brock & B.M. Taylor (eds.) *The First R: Every Child's Right to Read* (p. 133-159), Teachers College Press, Newark: DE.

Turner, J. C. (1995) The influence of classroom contexts on young children's motivation for literacy. Reading Research Quarterly, 30, 410-441.

Van Galen, G.P., (1991). Handwriting: Issues for a psychomotor theory. *Human Movement Science,* 10, 165-191.

Wolf, M., (1999). What time may tell: Towards a new conceptualization of developmental dyslexia. *Annals of Dyslexia,* 49, 3-23.

Zimmerman, B. and Riesemberg, R. (1997). Becoming a self-regulated writer: A social-cognitive perspective. *Contemporary Educational Psychology.*

Steven G. Feifer, Ed.S., NCSP    Philip A. De Fina, Ph.D., ABPdN